The Burgundy Journey:
Using Hope, Humor & Faith to
Conquer Adversity. No Matter What

Table of Contents:

Preface

Dedication

Preface

I called this book The Burgundy Journey because the awareness ribbon for Antiphospholipid Syndrome, or APS is burgundy. Having hope, humor, and faith no matter what, is really central to this whole struggle. You will see just how important those things are when you get further into the book. As you read my story, I hope you take with you the daily struggles that I, and others like me, with multiple disabilities, face each day. Because we don't look outwardly sick, many people believe that it's all in our heads. It is not. APS is sometimes referred to as an invisible disease because you can't see it on the outside, but it is real on the inside. I never thought that I would write this kind of book, or any other book for that matter, but I needed to share my story. As you will see with the backstory I provide, I have had a lot of adversity and a lot of strong willed people with me throughout my journey. When people tell me "you look good" or "you don't look sick," I sometimes want to scream at them: "if you only knew what was going on inside my body as it is being ravaged by this incurable disease, you may think differently." I know they are trying to help, but sometimes it just doesn't. When I tell people that I'm exhausted, they say "me too." It's not that kind of tired. It is complete and total exhaustion, not a tired exhaustion that "normal" people get. As for the memory loss, it's the same thing. I literally cannot remember certain things from minute to minute. Pen and paper have become my constant friend now! I hope that by telling my personal story and the adversities and hardships I have had to overcome, will inspire others to look at their lives and think how lucky they are to be where they are in this world. Remember that no one is promised tomorrow, nor are we promised the next minute. I have chosen to remain strong and fight for what I believe is best for myself and my son. Even when there are days that I want to give up, I know I can't. I have never been a quitter, and I'm not about to start now. I have tried to live my life by doing the right thing, and have decided that I will face this struggle head on, using hope, humor, and faith. God has chosen me to be the one to tell you about this often misdiagnosed and misunderstood disease. Whether or not you choose to listen is your prerogative. Never give up, never lose faith, and most importantly, keep a sense of humor about things. It really does help. Now, as you read my story, please think about what you would do when faced with such difficult circumstances. Will you be the one to run away or will you be the one that is going to face things head on? Will you be outraged by what has happened or will you just stand by and not do anything at all? Look deep into yourself to find the answers.

Dedication

This book is dedicated to my Mom and my sister who both taught me to live every day to the fullest. Thank you for your love and guidance throughout my life. I would not be where I am today without your constant and unwavering belief in me. Even in the face of tragedy and adversity, you showed me how to be strong, fight until the end, laugh along the way, and never give up, no matter what. I love you both and miss you terribly each and every day.

1. Here Comes Trouble!

My story starts on May 29, 2008. Maybe not. Rewind to perhaps as far back as 2004. Up until May 28, 2008, life was just rolling along. Sure, there have been tragedies that had befallen me and my family, but little did I know my whole world, and life as I knew it, was about to change. ALOT. Let me give you a little background information here so we can get started and you can fully (maybe) understand the scope of what I have been dealing with since then.

July 31, 1969. Not a particularly memorable day unless of course, you are my parents. That's the day child number 5, girl number 3 arrives in the Champion family. That's right, me! Years later when I was growing up, Mom used to tell me I was her medical problem. Apparently, before I was even born, I was a "thyroid problem." Like I said, I was child number 5, so the signs and symptoms should have been easy to pick up on. When Mom wasn't feeling well, she went to her doctor, and he told her it was a "thyroid problem." She didn't realize she was pregnant, and about 9 months later, the "thyroid problem" was born! As Mom told me later, at 2 weeks old I had pneumonia. The doctor had never treated someone so young, and to top it all off, how in the world do you get pneumonia in August? Should have known then that I was going to be trouble!

Growing up the youngest of 5 was not always easy, but it was always eventful! My childhood was not one of great monetary wealth, but the love my Mom had for us was worth more than anything money could buy. She was always there for us. There was my oldest sister Elaine, who was 14 years older than me. Next came my brother John, who is 12 years older, my sister Martha Sue (Mart), who is 6 years older, and finally my brother Vernon, who is 4 years older than me. Whether it was soccer, baseball, band, delivering the weekly newspaper or getting my oldest sister to and from college just about every weekend, Mom was our taxi driver. I was the first girl to play for our little league team way back when, and for a brief while, my Dad was the coach. Mom also made sure that Cub Scouts, Boy Scouts, Brownies and Girl Scouts were covered. When we got jobs, she would drive us until we got our license and our own cars. She even went with me when I had a college class at night and was afraid to go there alone. She would sit and read for the 2 hours I was in class. She joked that she was now college educated, even though she had never gotten to finish high school. She also was the nurse who took us to doctors appointments and the more than occasional hospital E R visit. Usually that was my older brother Vernon or yours truly who had managed to break or sprain something. If one of us was sick in the middle of the night, Mom was the one who sat with us until the fever broke, the puking stopped or we finally just fell asleep. You will see later why this was so important, and how we sometimes took for granted that she would always be around to guide us. She truly was the strongest, funniest, and most positive person I have ever met. She was the glue that held this family together on more than one occasion when things seemed lost.

I won't bore you with the everyday hustle and bustle of my childhood, but suffice to say, it was always an adventure. I'm going to skip through all that and get to the real reasons I wrote this book. A number of very important, very traumatic events helped shape my life and I would like to share them with you now.

My cousin Staci & I. I'm on the right

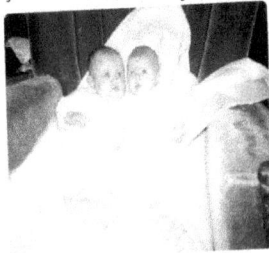

Mom & I

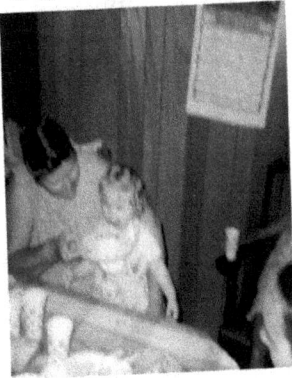

Me at 1 year old

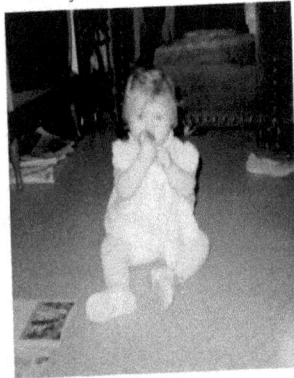

The Champion Siblings: John, Elaine, Vernon, Me & Mart

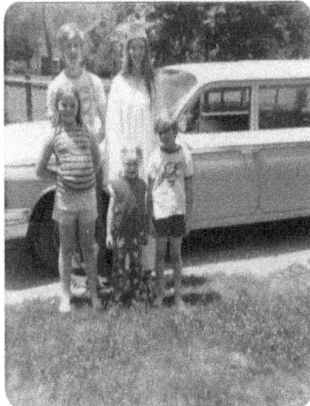

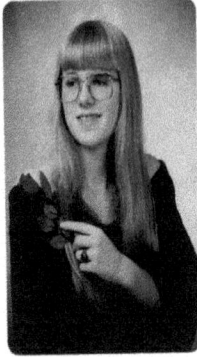

High School graduation 1987

College graduation 1989

College graduation 1991

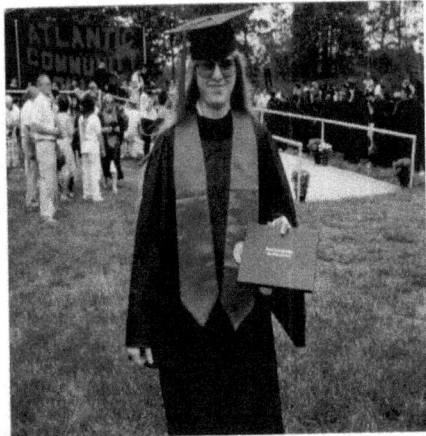

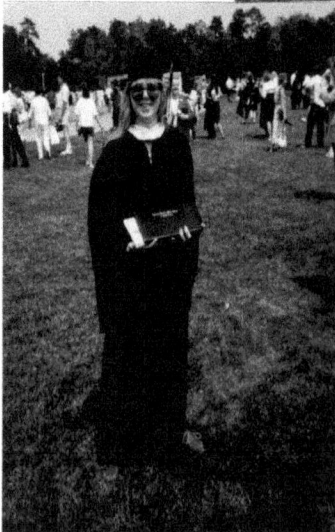

2. Tragedy Part 1

In early 1986, my life was about to change dramatically. Elaine was diagnosed at age 30 with breast cancer. I remember thinking, this can't be. By the time she was diagnosed, we were told that she wouldn't live out the weekend. When Mom asked her if she had noticed any signs or symptoms, she admitted that she had for about the past 6 months to a year. She didn't tell anybody because she didn't want to worry us and besides, she was a second grade teacher at the very same school we had all attended and didn't think it would be fair to her students if she couldn't teach them what they needed to learn. She was always active and enjoyed not only teaching those students, but she was young and had her whole life ahead of her. She had traveled the world with her best friend since childhood, Holly. They went to Rome, London, Paris, and Athens. She loved to travel and explore and most of all, she loved to learn new things. That is the knowledge she brought back to share with her students. Mind you though, she couldn't read a map to save her life! I witnessed this first hand on many a trip that Elaine, Mom, my siblings and I went on. None is more memorable than the trip to Washington D C. My Mom was the designated map reader for obvious reasons, and kept telling Elaine to make a right when we got to a certain road. Every time we would approach the road, Elaine would make a left! This happened at least a half a dozen times before she finally got it right! I can remember seeing the Washington Monument from the same angle every time. It was kind of nice to see it from a different angle when we finally got where we were going!

As the diagnosis became a reality, she fought as much as she could. The chemotherapy took its toll on her and I can remember her just throwing up constantly as she was receiving her dose. Her hair began falling out, and she began to lose weight. She was thin as it was, so losing weight was not good for her. I remember her joking one time that she wanted to lose some weight, but not like this! She continued to teach for a while, but the strain became too much. She battled for as long as she could and she had times when she was better, but not well. She spent a lot of time in the hospital, but she did prove the doctors wrong about not living out the weekend. By this point, the cancer had spread to her bones so she had a hard time walking. My Mom was right there by her side the whole time. She would go to work and as soon as she got done, she would go straight to the hospital. There was many a night that she slept there, and towards the end, the nurses made sure the bed next to my sister was empty so Mom would have somewhere to sleep. As my high school graduation approached in 1987, I remember Elaine crying and I asked her what was wrong. She said that she was sad because she wouldn't be able to keep her promise to me about taking me to Rome for my graduation. I looked at her and told her I didn't care about that and if it was meant to be, I would get there someday. All I wanted was her at my graduation. Her and I were the closest of the five of us, maybe because she was the oldest and wanted to make sure I was protected and taken care of. She did make my graduation, and I was the happiest person in the world. Several months before her death, she needed back surgery to relieve the pressure from a pinched nerve. When she didn't start to improve after a few days, we, and the nurses, suspected something was wrong. Come to find out that when the doctor was operating, he slipped and severed another nerve, making her bedridden for the remainder of her life. He never told anyone about that, and we found out accidentally when Elaine's primary doctor mentioned it. We all watched the beginning of the end, and I remember thinking how tragic it was to see someone so vibrant and young go to basically being an invalid in a year's time. My heart was, and continues to be, broken.

Her sad tragic journey came to an end on March 24, 1988. She was 32. My Mom, sister and I were with her when she died. Dad and my brothers arrived shortly after she passed.

It was a blessing for her, but for me it was a feeling of overwhelming grief and sorrow. I had never experienced the death of someone I loved so much. John had the task of calling our aunts and uncles to tell them the news. It was the first time I had ever seen him cry (well, unless you count the time Mart "fixed" his broken nose. That was hysterical for us, but not for him!). Shortly after her death, our pastor, who was coming for his daily visit, and had no idea that she had just died, overheard a doctor arguing with the nurses at the desk. He was saying things like "why do I have to be the one to tell them?" and "I didn't even know the patient or her family." The nurse told him it was because he had been left in charge by the patient's primary doctor when he went on vacation the previous week. She also told him that he had failed to answer any pages from the nurses and requests from the family to speak with him. After our pastor found out who the doctor was talking about, he told my parents that he had never wanted to punch somebody in the face as much as he did in that moment! The doctor finally came in and took one quick look at Elaine and put his head down as he left the room mumbling to us "I'm sorry, there's nothing I can do." The nurse was actually the one to pronounce her dead. We found out that the doctor tragically lost his own son in the September 11th attacks on the World Trade Center. I hope whoever was given the task of telling him the news was able to do so with more finesse than he was capable of. This doctor has since died also.

As word spread that Elaine had died, the love and support of the community was overwhelming. We began planning her funeral, and those next few days were excruciatingly painful for me. As I said, I had never had to bury someone who I had loved so much. My Mom was devastated, not only that she had lost her child, but because it brought back memories for her about burying her younger sister who had died in the 1960's.She too had breast cancer and was I believe 30 or 31 when she died. I wasn't even a twinkle in Mom and Dad's eyes when my aunt died, but later on in life I would find out about a very important connection we would have.

The days had finally come to say our last goodbyes to a beautiful, young life that had been taken way too soon. We had a viewing the night before the funeral, and then again on the day of. The line of people was never ending. Friends, family, students and former students, school coworkers and administrators, politician friends of my father, young and old, came to pay their respects to her. It truly was exhausting for all of us, but it just proved how special and loved Elaine really was. The funeral was now over, and we went to her casket one final time. I remember my father saying, "Don't say goodbye, say I'll see you later." That's what I did. Even today when I visit her grave, I don't say "goodbye" but rather "see you later." I love you little one, and always will. I don't know why, but I called her little one. Kind of ironic because she was the older one. Even today when I see certain things or smell certain kinds of foods, I think of her.

After Elaine's death, the media center at the school was renamed in her memory so that those who knew her and those who didn't could be reminded of the positive impact she had on so many students lives. What a fitting tribute to her. As that sad chapter in life closed, more was yet to come. Some things were happy, others not so much.

About 9 months later, we welcomed the first Champion grandchild to the clan. Anna Rebecca was born on December 13, 1988. John and his wife Joanne named her after Joanne's grandmother and decided to give her Elaine's middle name, Rebecca. What a joyous time for us.

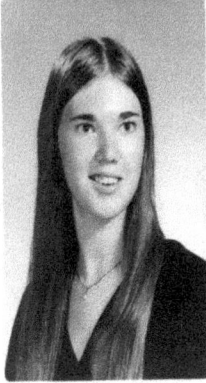
Elaine's high school graduation photo

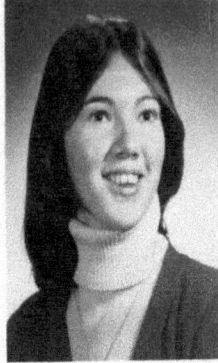
Elaine's college graduation photo

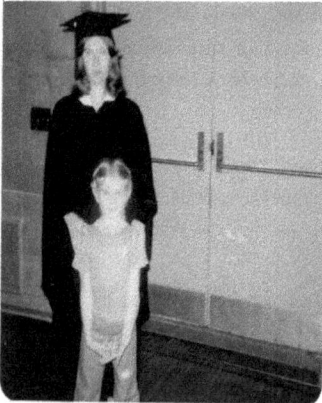
Elaine & I at Elaine's college graduation

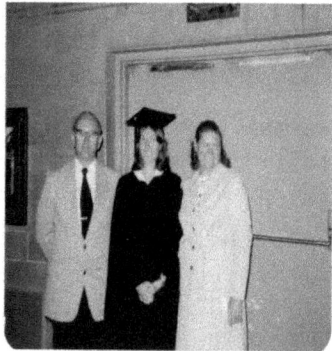
Dad, Elaine & Mom at Elaine's college graduation

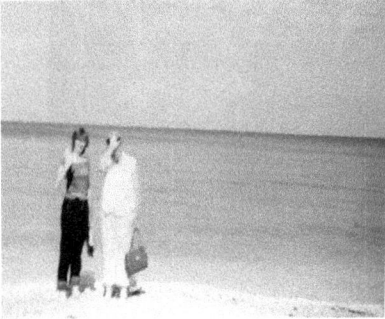

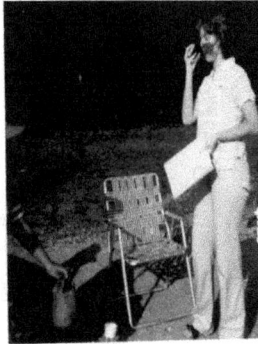

Elaine the scorekeeper

Elaine near the end

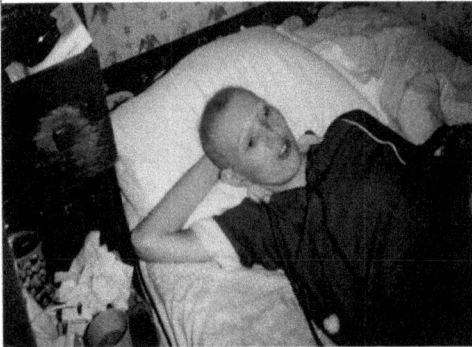

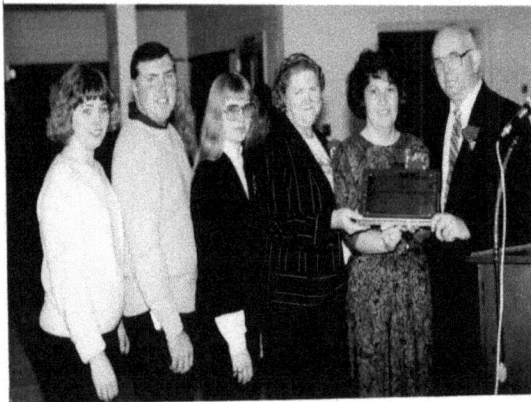

Mart, Vernon, Me, Mom, Holly & Dad at the ceremony naming the new school media center The Elaine P. Champion Media Center

3. Again?

April 8, 1990. Palm Sunday. We had just finished up our lunch when the fire department tone went off. Both Vernon and Dad are members. The call was for a car accident in front of the post office. We live about a mile or so from there, so off they go. Within 5 or 10 minutes, there is a knock on our door. Mom answers it, and standing there, is the chief of the rescue squad. He looks like the proverbial deer in the headlights. Mom says "Is it Vernon?" the chief says "No, it's John (my Dad)." That's all he said. With that, he hopped back into his truck and takes off. Mom, Mart, and I jumped in Mart's car and headed to the hospital. On our way there, we saw the medic unit coming in the opposite direction heading to the scene of the accident. She continued driving to the hospital, and when we got there, my Dad hadn't even been brought in yet, so we sat in the waiting room. When the medics finally arrived with Dad, things didn't look good. He had massive injuries. Shattered collarbone, a concussion, and multiple fractures in his leg, internal injuries, cuts, scrapes, and bruises. He had to have surgery. NOW. While we were escorted out to the waiting room again, the chief came in to tell us what had happened. My father is a fire policeman, so his job is to direct traffic at emergency scenes. While he was doing this at the scene of the original accident, one driver wasn't paying attention and hit him. The impact threw him up in to the air with such force, that when he landed he hit his head on the pavement and was clinically dead. Even though the rescue squad was on scene, it was not enough to help him. They knew it was bad. Things looked bleak. Guess they didn't know who they were dealing with though! My father is a stubborn man. He worked for several decades at a locally owned grocery store until they went out of business. He then went to work for the lottery department. In the 1970's and '80's, he was a politician. He served on the township committee and later served as mayor. After his days were done, he still participated in campaigns and political functions.

As we sat waiting for news, two men came in with a small child. We overheard them saying that they came to the hospital because some guy just walked out in front of them and he got hit. Little did we know at that point that this was the man responsible for putting my Dad in the hospital. The chief knew though and told the nurse to get them out of there before someone else got hurt. He didn't want them anywhere near us when he heard the driver blaming my Dad for this. We got moved to a more private area for everybody's safety. We waited and waited for hours for news. As people we knew began hearing about the accident, a few trickled in to support us. My poor mother. I can still see the tears in her eyes and the pain on her face. I imagine she was thinking that she had just buried her daughter two years ago, and now she may be burying her husband next. Dad made it through the surgery, but he was by no means out of the woods. If he survived, there would be the issue of the leg. The doctor was pretty sure Dad would never walk again. Also, what was the extent of the brain damage caused by the concussion? How about the broken collarbone? There were a lot of "what if's." When they finally put Dad in a room, we got to see the extent of the injuries. Mom stood over him and cried. We were all numb at this point. My Mom had such a look of pain and sadness about her, I just felt really bad for her. As the anesthesia wore off, Dad started having a reaction to it. He began kicking and screaming and tried to throw his casted leg over the side of the bed. The nurses and doctor asked Mom for permission to tie him down so he couldn't do more harm to himself or the people around him. As painful as it was, Mom agreed. It was for the best. Again, Mom would begin spending all her waking, nonworking hours, at the hospital. She did come home at night as Dad progressed, but she knew there was a long road ahead of not only him, but her as well. Finally, after nearly 2 months in the hospital, Dad came home. Changes needed to be made, so Vernon and John built a ramp so Mom could push the wheelchair up and down without having to lift Dad. Dad was the main source of income, so things were a little tight, but Mom just faced the challenge head on and kept her smile and positive attitude. There were countless hours of physical therapy, and finally Dad was able to use a walker. The doctor who had told us he would never walk again was told by my Dad that he had to walk because Mart was getting married in June, and he had to walk his daughter down the aisle. Guess what? Mart's wedding day came and Dad walked her down the aisle. There was not a dry eye in the church. See I told you he is stubborn!

The person responsible for nearly killing my father finally had his day in court. The judge looked at him and said "weren't you in my courtroom recently for drug possession?" The public defender immediately objected, even though it was true. It felt like a slap in the face to my parents when the judge told the guy that he understood that he had small children and it was near Christmas, so he gave him until after the New Year to pay. He laughed all the way out of the courtroom and my parents never saw a dime. Had he been put in jail when he was convicted of the drug offenses, perhaps my Dad would not have been nearly killed. Perhaps the next victim of this vile human being might still be alive too. You see, shortly after he laughed his way out of the courtroom, he went on to do the most unspeakable, heinous crime imaginable. He raped and killed a young teenage girl. Karma got him back though because a few years later, after being convicted of the rape and murder, he died in jail of AIDS. A fitting end to this monster's life.

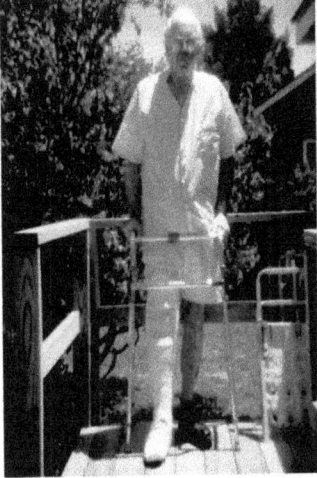

Photos of Dad after his accident

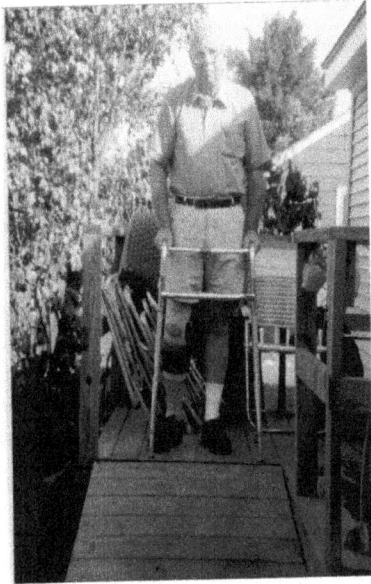

4. Finally, Some Good News!

On December 12, 1992, Mart and her husband Don welcomed their first child to the world, Stephanie Michelle. They would go on to have two more children; Frances Elaine (named after both her grandmothers) was born on June 15, 1995. James John (or JJ as we call him, named after both his grandfathers) was born on October 13, 1997.

Things were looking up at that point, and more was about to come. It was July of 1994, and I had been invited to a friend's wedding. I wasn't dating anyone at that point, so I went alone.

When I got to the reception, I was seated at a table with people who I absolutely had no clue who they were. They were apparently college friends of the bride and groom, but that didn't help me! I am not a really social person if I don't know you, so it was kind of hard for me not knowing anybody at the table. The couples were either married or engaged, so that left me out of the loop. There was one guy there who was about at bored and nervous as I was, because he too had come by himself. We began talking and later danced. I was just being polite, as I had no intention of getting involved with anyone at that point. Then as I was getting ready to leave, I did something that I would never have dreamed of doing. I told him that if he wanted to talk to me, the happy couple had my number. I left it at that.

5. Some Guy Named Keith

A few weeks had passed, and I got a phone call from, who I thought was my former boss, Keith, who had recently lost his wife at a young age to cancer. I had told him that if he needed to talk or anything, I was there for him. After dealing with Elaine's death at such a young age, I thought maybe I could help him with his wife's death from cancer too. I just wanted to offer the hand of friendship. Only problem was, the Keith on the phone wasn't my former boss; it was THE Keith from the wedding! UMM, can you say awkward! I don't even think the Keith on the phone realized what I was talking about when I asked him how he was doing and if he needed anything. Anyway, when I got myself out of that predicament, Keith and I had a nice conversation. He told me that he had waited until his friend had come back from the honeymoon to ask him for my number, so that is why it took him so long to call me. We agreed to go out and on the first date we took our now mutual friends with us just to be safe.

We began dating and in June 1995, right there on the mini golf course, he got down on one knee and proposed. I was shocked! I tell people that the best thing that happened that night was that immediately after the proposal I got a hole in one! Mart jokes about it too because she was close to her due date with Fran, and that kid just didn't want to come out. She said that Keith finally popping the question sent her into labor. About a week later, Fran was born.

We had decided on the following September for the wedding. Of course being the Type A personality that I am, I got started right away planning every little detail down to the last miniscule item. I had told my parents that rather than them going into debt trying to pay for the whole thing, that since I had a job I would pay for everything except for the reception. They agreed and so that's how we did it. Thank goodness Mart was there too. She helped me plan and some of the things I did were just like the things she had done for her own wedding. I took Mom and Mart with me dress shopping. I don't own any dresses, not my style, so picking one out for the most important day of my life was not going to be easy. When we walked into the first bridal shop, the saleswoman asked what I was looking for. Mart, knowing me all too well, told her that I wasn't a frilly or fancy type of girl. It was kind of funny because I thought this was going to be a nightmare picking out a dress knowing that I would wear it one time and be done with it. Turns out that the very first dress I tried on I liked and bought it. Dress-check! Now it was time to concentrate on the flowers. I had decided on teal for my bridesmaids dresses. Again, Mart was right there to help. As a matter of fact, she made all of the flowers for everybody involved. She made my bouquet and one for me to throw. She also made all of the centerpieces for the tables. It was no easy task, so thank goodness she is crafty! Flowers-check!

We needed to figure out where the reception was going to be held, because Keith and I both have huge families. There were about 300 on the guest list including family and friends. My father and brother are both firemen as mentioned before, so we were able to secure a fire hall that held over 300 people and because they are firemen, we got it at a reduced rate. Reception hall-check!

Things seemed to be falling into place, but one big issue remained. Keith was raised a strict Catholic, and I was raised Methodist. I knew that I wanted to get married in my church, and Keith had no problem with it. I was willing to have a priest there as kind of a co minister so that he could feel as though he was still faithful to his upbringing. We went to meet the priest who we thought would do it, but as soon as we got there, this guy starts out with " Dorothy you have to...go to Catholic classes, you have to...let me do the ceremony, you have to...promise to raise the children Catholic." WRONG THING TO SAY TO ME! Nobody tells me that I "have to..." basically give up MY religion to satisfy a certain family member who wanted the whole ceremony done Catholic because they felt if it wasn't done that way then the marriage wouldn't be legal in the eyes of God. Bye bye priest. We ended up doing it with just my Methodist minister.

As the date got closer and closer, there seemed to be more and more interference from family (his, not mine). Seemed like no matter what we wanted, it wasn't good enough for them. As a matter of fact, I have to laugh at this now, but it wasn't funny at the time. When Keith's mother found out that we were not serving alcohol at the reception, she actually invited ALL of Keith's side of the family back to our house afterwards so they could drink there. First of all, neither Keith nor I drink. None of my family drinks. We couldn't see shelling out a ton of money on something that neither one of us does. Just because his family drinks all the time, does not mean that we should go broke feeding their habit. Secondly, if we weren't having alcohol at the reception, what makes you think that we would allow you to get drunk in OUR house on OUR wedding night?? Needless to say, the idea of them coming back to the house was stopped immediately. Also, there was a day, about a week before the wedding, that his mother called my mother and began yelling at her about me not helping Keith with the housework, the bills, etc. I was not living in the house yet, so those things were not my responsibility. Keith knew that and I knew that. We had decided that when we finally did get married, I would take over those things. This was the last straw. NOBODY, and I mean NOBODY, attacks my mother like that. She told Keith's mother that whatever the problem was between her and us, that we would have to settle because she was not getting involved. I left my house and went to my soon to be home. When I got there, needless to say, things got really ugly. Without going into the details, it ended with Keith rocking in the corner, and his mother being carried to the car by his father. I was just a tad bit upset!

The final week came and all the final preparations were being made. I had people on high alert for anything suspicious at the ceremony. They knew what to do!

Finally, on September 21, 1996, we became Mr. and Mrs. Keith Smaniotto. Everything went off without a hitch, but it just so happened that it was about 90 degrees that day, so I was sweating from the heat! My girls were fanning me to keep me cool. After the wedding and reception, we were ready to go to OUR new home. As we approached it, there was an accident so we got detoured around another way. We weren't really familiar with the area yet, so Keith, still dressed in his tuxedo, got out of the car and asked for directions (first and last time he's ever asked for directions!). The fireman looked in the car and saw me still in my gown, and must have thought, man, I've got to get this guy home ,it's his wedding night! He led us through and we made it home. When we got there, we had no electric, but that really didn't matter! We left the next day on our honeymoon to London. The city was nice, but the food, not so much. I couldn't wait to get home and have some real food. I'm just not a kidney pie kind of girl!

As we settled in as husband and wife, we began talking about starting a family. We both wanted to wait at least a year before we started trying. As we approached our first anniversary, we were thinking about traveling again. Keith suggested Rome, knowing that Elaine had wanted to take me there before she died. See Elaine, I told you if it was meant to be I would see Rome someday. We began planning our adventure, and shortly before we left, I found out I was pregnant. I wanted to tell Keith in a special way, so I decided to get a book with Italian phrases in it. The premise, I told him was to learn just a little Italian in case we needed it. He can speak some Italian since that is his heritage, but not me. I pointed out a phrase to him that was something to the effect of I need a doctor. I used the positive pregnancy test to point to the saying. It took him a couple of minutes to realize what I was doing, but once he did he was excited. We were going to be parents! We went on our anniversary trip, and a couple of days in I got sick. I knew it had to be a sinus infection because the city of Rome is so dirty, it is hard to breathe. I called Mart from Rome, and at first she didn't even recognize my voice because I was so sick! She was working for an OB GYN at the time, so I figured she'd know what to do. She told me to find a doctor there and explain the situation. I wasn't about to take a chance with an unborn child, so we decided to cut our trip short and return home so I could get help. Bear in mind that this was in the days before 9/11, so things weren't as tough as they are now. We went to the airport and told the airline that we needed to fly home now. They asked why, and I told them that I was pregnant and needed to get home to seek medical attention. I expected them to charge us an arm and a leg to change our flight, but they just looked at me and said get on the plane. They waved us through and we were homeward bound. We got home, and sure enough, it was a sinus infection. I got treated for it and things were good. Then next 7 months seemed to pass quickly, with really no real problems to report. I did have a couple of weird cravings though. Pineapple and gummy cola bottles. Yeah, I don't know why! As my due date approached, it seemed as though this kid did not want to come out. Finally, four days after my due date, I was about to become a Mommy!

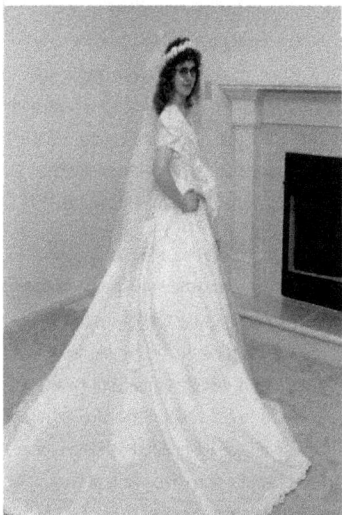
Me on my wedding day

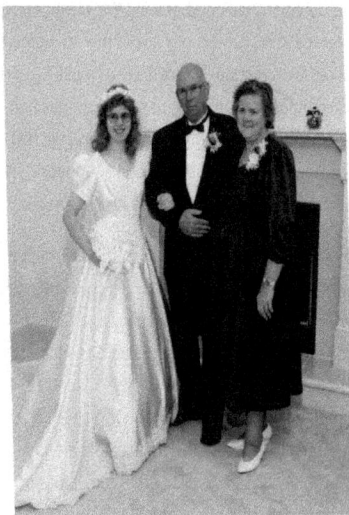
Me, Dad & Mom on my wedding day

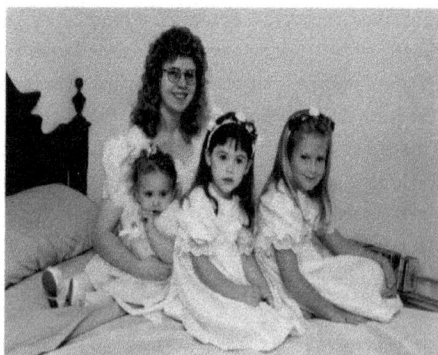
Me with my nieces Fran, Steph, & Anna on my wedding day

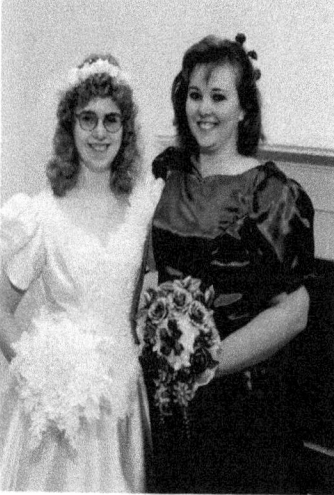
Me with Mari on my wedding day

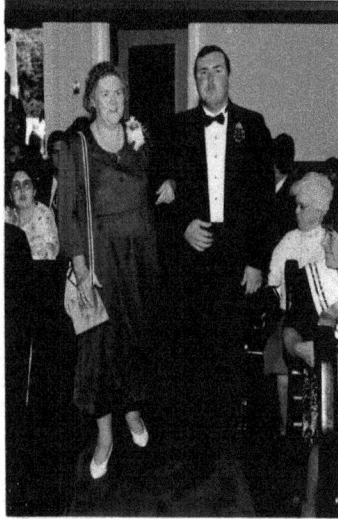
Vernon walking Mom down the aisle on my wedding day

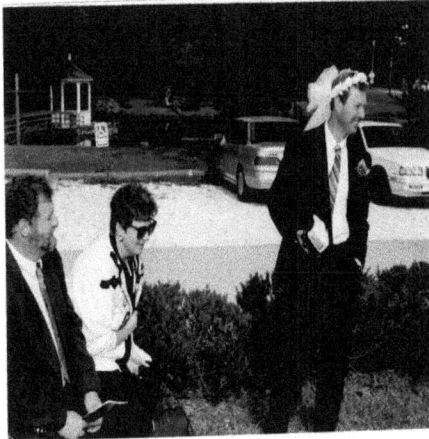
My brother John keeping an eye on my veil for me on my wedding day

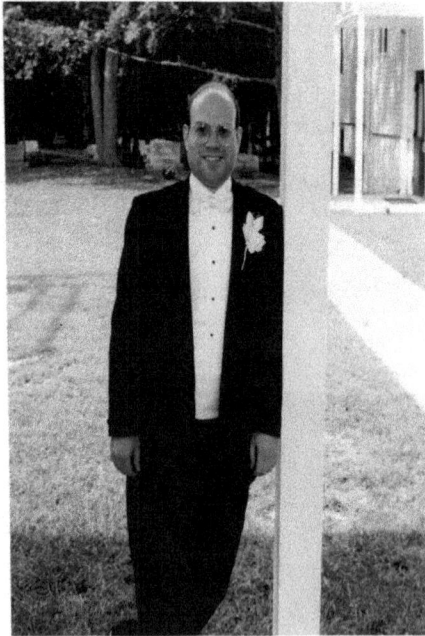

keith on our wedding day

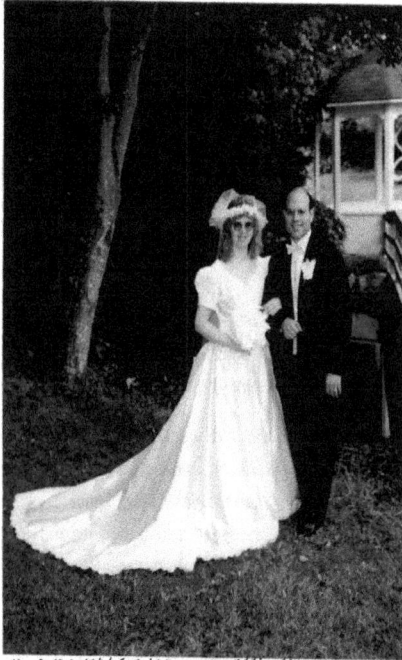

Mr. & Mrs. Keith Smaniotto on our wedding day

My family on our wedding day. Vernon, John, Joanne, Mom, Keith, Me, Dad, Mart, Fran, Don, Steph, & Anna

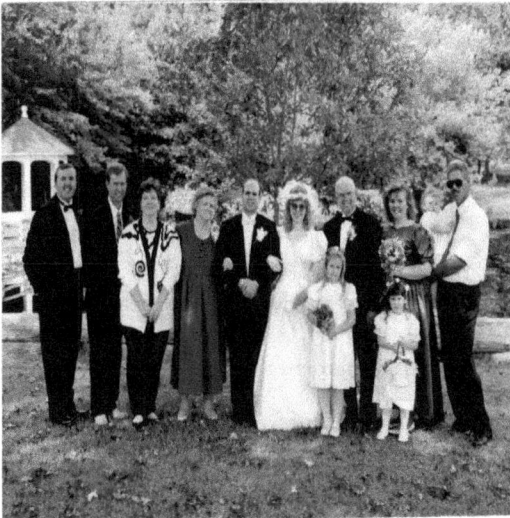

6. My Reason For Being

On June 27, 1998, at 12:21 AM, Alexander Keith Smaniotto makes his grand entrance into the world. He is 6 lbs. 11 oz. and 19 ¾" long. He is beautiful. Just after he was born, though joy turned to fear. As he was being born, he suffered something called pneumothorax-holes in his lungs. I didn't know what was going on and had no idea if he would be alright. He was whisked away just as quickly as he had arrived. The odd thing was we were told that his APGAR scores were all 10's. He was immediately put in an incubator and hooked up to all kinds of wires and machines.

Keith and I began calling our parents to let them know we had a boy. Those words were met with "A boy?" See, seems as though everyone thought for sure I was having a girl! None the less, the new grandparents were happy. They would come down later in the day to meet him.

The nurses came in and told us that Alex would need to be moved to a hospital about an hour and a half away because he was going to need special treatment in a neonatal ICU. My heart sank. I kept thinking that I couldn't lose this baby. I hadn't even held my little boy yet. Arrangements were made to bring the specialized ambulance and neonatologist down to get him. By this time, it was late morning and the grandparents, aunts and uncles had begun to arrive to meet the newest member of the family. They had no idea that any of this was going on, so when they got there, it was a shock for them. I was finally able to get out of bed and walk down to the nursery. This was the first time I had seen him since he was whisked away. It broke my heart to see him hooked up to all kinds of tubes, wires, and machines. The nurses let me hold him for the first time. I cried. As we waited for the specialist to arrive, my father wanted to pray around the incubator, so we did.

The neonatologist had arrived, and went in to examine Alex. She came out shaking her head. Seems as though somehow the pneumothorax had resolved itself. She said it would do more harm than good to move him at this point, so he stayed right where he was. The power of prayer! He began to get stronger and stronger, and even tried to lift his little day old head off of the blanket by himself.

I was discharged the next day, but Alex had to stay. Again, my heart was broken. I didn't want to leave him. The nurses assured me that I could call and check on him and that I could come back the next day to see him. I left the hospital empty handed. That night, I didn't sleep at all. I kept thinking how am I going to make it through the night knowing that I am not there for my baby. I think I called the nurses about 6 times that night. Each time they were nice and told me that he was holding his own and improving with each breath. The next morning we got a call saying we could bring him home. I couldn't get there fast enough to do that. We brought him home and were now ready to begin life as a family.

He was having some problems adjusting to formula, so we had to get him a special kind. Seemed like everything upset his stomach and made him throw up. He was about 2 weeks old at this point, and in the middle of the night he just wouldn't stop fussing. I called the pediatrician, and he said to give him a tiny bit of plain antacid and bring him to the office in the morning. I did what I was told, and within minutes, he began to vomit uncontrollably. He stopped and went limp in my arms. I screamed at him not to leave me and to come back to me. Keith was on the phone with 911 at this point, and even though they got there within 5 minutes, it seemed like hours. I rode in the ambulance with him and Keith followed in the car. When we got to the hospital, he was hooked up to all kinds of machines again, and again, my heart was breaking. I refused to leave his side. I had to leave it once before, and I was not about to do it again. I wasn't leaving without him. Once he was stabilized, the doctors had asked what we gave him. I told him about the call to the pediatrician, and about the antacid. Then it dawned on me. What if the "plain" antacid was actually mint flavored? You see, I am allergic to mint and maybe Alex was too. Sure enough, when you look at the label, it says there is mint flavoring. Turns out it was a severe allergic reaction. I will NOT make that mistake again. As a precaution, the pediatrician wanted to send him home with a monitor just to be sure nothing else was happening. Keith is Epileptic, so they had to rule that out too. Alex wore the monitor 24/7 for 2 months. It did go off a couple of times, but only because a lead got knocked off or crimped. We also found out that he had a case of reflux, so we had to add cereal to his formula quite early in his life.

As he grew, we began to plan his Christening. He was still wearing the monitor, but the doctor told us we could remove it for that. Good thing. Could you imagine him getting water on him and then getting zapped? He began to get stronger and stronger, but a new problem developed. Ear infections. Constantly. His little ears hurt so much that he screamed every time we tried to lay him down. We had been told to put a pillow under the mattress to elevate it, but that did little to help. This went on from the age of about 6 months to age 18 months. There were times when I would sit down in a beach lounge chair at night and hold him on my chest all night long just so he and I could get some sleep. There was a stretch of about 2 weeks where I did that and didn't sleep a wink. My boss looked at me and told me I looked like I was about to fall over from lack of sleep. I really think it would have happened if we weren't able to get him to a pediatric ear nose and throat specialist. Finally, in December 1999, he had ear tubes placed and has been fine ever since. The problems with his ears did not stop his speech from developing though.

I remember one day when he was about 6 months old, shortly before he began having all the ear infections, I had laid him down for a nap. I went downstairs to try and get some work done while he was asleep. Next thing I know I hear "Ma, I'm crying!" I had no idea where it had come from because I didn't have the TV or radio on. I went upstairs to find Alex, fresh off his nap, smiling at me and holding onto the side of his crib. Again, the words came "Ma, I'm crying!" I was stunned! Here he is, 6 months old, and speaking in complete sentences. I should have known then that this was no ordinary child. As the months progressed, even with all the problems with his ears, he began to advance by leaps and bounds. He would do things that most kids that age would start doing until they were 3 or 4 years old or older. I read to him every night and he seemed to hang on every word of the story. When he got fussy, we would put on some Motown music or some oldies, and he would calm down. We thought he was just a bright kid, but looking back, some things now click that should have made us realize just how special he really is. At about a year to 18 months of age, he became obsessed with cars. Not just the car goes "vroom vroom", but "that is a Chevy Silverado, that's a Ford Explorer, a Dodge Ram," etc. He could tell you make and model of any car you put in front of him. People at our church were amazed, and there was many a time that we would be going to or coming from church and they would stop him in the parking lot, point to a car, and wait for his response. He always got it right. By the time he was 2 years old, he could read. Not just "cat" and "dog "read, but really read. He took his favorite book to Sunday School one day and read it to his teacher. She was floored. I still remember it "Wendell Gets Dressed". We still have it. At the age of 3, he began playing some learning games on the computer. He also began to speak Japanese. This was a mystery to us because no one we knew spoke another language, let alone Japanese. He continued to flourish, and could have an adult conversation with you and understand what you were telling him. He taught us more about dinosaurs, cars, Spiderman, and a host of other subjects than I ever could dream about knowing. He also loved any and all things related to Egypt. King Tut, the pyramids, the Nile and whatever else he could find that related to ancient Egypt. He would give you not just an overview of his particular subject, but in depth details. Vernon used to jokingly argue with him because for a time he swore his name was "Albert Jack." Vernon would say, "No, it's Alex." Alex would say "No, it's Albert Jack." Wonder what Albert Einstein's middle name was? In this time frame, he also developed a few little obsessions, not that that is necessarily a bad thing. He hated the color blue. Don't buy anything that was blue or else he would have a meltdown. He would tell you how things were, good or bad. He was brutally honest (Still is. Again, not a bad thing). He would need all of his toys lined up just so, and don't even think about moving them the slightest bit out of line. This was cause for a meltdown. He developed a love of Penny Loafers, and to this day he still wears them. He says they are comfortable, so why fight it. The shoes make the boy! People notice if he's NOT wearing them more than if he is wearing them. The loafers are a part of him and a good part I might add. My advice is pick your battles carefully and don't sweat the small things.

Alex and my Mom are like soul mates. He loves her, she loves him, and they both have a contagious smile and laugh. She calls him " Grandmom's Angel." He hugs her tightly in return. He is 4 now, so he's still a little young to understand what is about to happen. Without going too in depth in this chapter, I'll touch on it a go back to it in the next chapter. Mom had been sick on and off for about 4 years. She came to live with us and sadly, passed away at our house. On the day she died, she hugged him, told him that she loved him, and he told her that he loved her. It would be the last time they spoke to each other. When we had to break the news to him, we knew we had to do it right because this was not a "normal" 4 year old. We told him she had died, and his response was "she's living with Jesus now." That's how he saw it and that got him through it.

A few months later, it was time to start thinking about sending him to school. We filled out the paperwork, and during the summer they had the kindergarten roundup where they test the kids to see what they already know. When it was Alex's turn, the teacher took him into a room and asked him his shapes, colors, name, etc. When she came out, she said to us "I have to tell you, I've never had a child read me the names of the crayon colors while drawing." He was telling her that it was sunflower yellow, fire engine red, violet purple, etc. She continued with "he knows all the letters of the alphabet, his shapes, and how to spell his name. He's like a little professor, very advanced for his age." Remember that phrase "little professor."

September rolls around and it's the first day of school. He does his thing and comes home. As the year progresses, I get a phone call one day from his teacher. She's half laughing but kind of serious. She says "I have to tell you something about Alex." Uh oh I think. "He told me that I wrote my "r" wrong on the board." This woman has been a teacher for probably 20 years or so, and here's a 5 year old boy telling her she wrote her "r" wrong. I apologized to her, but she laughed because she said "he was right. The way the letter was written on paper looked different than the way I wrote it on the board." The year progresses, and by now there is a full time substitute in the class because the other teacher has had a number of family and personal tragedies and will be out for most of the year. I get to know the new teacher pretty well, and her and I still speak every once in a while. It's now Christmas time and I go in for the classroom party. The teacher pulls me aside and says "I have to tell you something about Alex." Again I think uh oh. She says that while the other children were doing their craft, Alex was reading the newspaper that had been put down to keep the desks clean! I didn't want to ask him about it at the party, so on the ride home I asked him how his day went before I got there. He thinks for a minute and then says "Mom, who is George Will?" I nearly drove off the road! I explained who he was, then Alex asks, "well then, what does Congress do?" Boy is that a loaded question! He finishes out his kindergarten year and prepares for first grade.

First grade rolls around, and it just so happens that the sub from kindergarten got a full time job as a first grade teacher. Alex, at my request, was placed in her room. Things were a bit bumpy, but there were several children in the room with differing disabilities. Then one night in January of 2005, she called me from home. She said she was concerned about Alex's behavior. Little things that most kids wouldn't even notice bothered him. The ticking of the clock, the lighting, the noise, the texture of his clothes and the tags inside his shirt really seemed to be a problem for him. He also couldn't stand to have things out of place and if he made a mistake, he would just totally have a breakdown. She suggested that we maybe take him to a therapist to see what was going on. I knew the loss of my Mom was very hard for him even at a very young age. Maybe that was it.

I made an appointment, and within a few sessions, the therapist gave me news that I was not prepared for. After watching him and his behaviors, she told me that he had something called Asperger's Syndrome. I had no idea what that was. She explained that Asperger's Syndrome is a form of Autism commonly referred to as High Functioning Autism because the child has extreme intelligence, but lacks the social skills to deal with outside distractions. She explained that things like ticking clocks, lighting, noise, texture ,color aversion, and a million other things that other people can filter out, Asperger's kids can't. Everything started to fall into place. Remember the vast knowledge of cars? How about dinosaurs and Spiderman? The lining up of the toys? What about those penny loafers? All are signs of Asperger's. She told us that many times, children are referred to as "little professors." I told you to remember that phrase. When my head stopped spinning, I asked her what we could do. She said we would have to teach Alex how to deal with and control those outside forces. At first, the only other people besides myself and Keith that knew were his teacher and the special ed department at school. Keith wanted to know how this could happen, and did it come from one of us. I still didn't have an answer, so I couldn't tell him. I went out and got my hands on any book I could related to Asperger's and Autism, and I think I read about 20 books within 2 weeks. I wanted to know everything I could to help my son. This was not going to be an easy journey, but I was determined to help my son get whatever he needed to succeed. We eventually told our families, and of course my family was very supportive. They told me that whatever I needed, they would be there for us. Mart is a special ed teacher, so she understood. Vernon, even though he has no kids of his own, loves his nieces and nephews unconditionally. He is the one person who Alex and I can go to in a time of need and he talks Alex through the problem or issue. Keith's family was not as accepting at first, partly because they have never had to deal with something like this. They don't really understand the quirks and details of the disease, and I think they look at it as a failure to their family because we don't have a perfect child. Guess what? Alex is perfect to us. I know that they will probably be mad at me for some of the things I have said, but when Keith and I look at the differences in the way each side of the family has dealt with it, my family has been there for us, no questions asked and has supported and loved him unconditionally. I think this is due to the way Keith and I were brought up. We were raised very differently, and that has shown throughout this whole journey. We decided not to tell Alex right away, because we didn't want him to think that he was different and couldn't do certain things. It was hard for me to keep his condition from him because he is so smart and can usually figure out if something is up. Finally one night I kneeled down to his level and began to cry. He asked me why I was crying, and I told him I needed to tell him something about himself. I told him that he had something called "Asperger's Syndrome," and he looked at me and said "is that why I'm not like the other kids?" I cried some more and told him yes. As he began to accept and live with this, he said to me one day "You know Mom, I find my Asperger's a blessing, not a disability." I knew then that he would be alright.

Now comes the fun part! Now that Alex was "classified" as a special ed student, we had to get the paperwork to back it up. We had to take him to a psychologist to be evaluated and confirm the diagnosis. Of course there are no doctors locally who can do this, according to the school, so we had to travel an hour and a half north to have it done. Ok, fine, done. Once the results came back, things start happening. I had to learn basically a whole new language with things called IEP's, CST's, best placement, and the list goes on.

Let's start with CST. Child Study Team. This is where things begin and end in the world of school special education terms. The CST is a group of people who are assembled to evaluate and help your child get the services they need and are entitled to in the educational setting. They work with you to help with placement and ideas about what they feel is best for your child. I think " great", someone to help all of us get through it. Maybe not. Next you have an IEP. Individual Education Plan. This is the plan they have for you, your child, and the teacher to follow to help the child succeed. Again, not. As first grade continued, things were a work in progress. The fear I had was that going into second grade, having a new teacher, and learning new rules, would really require effort on everyone's part. Second grade didn't go so well, but it was nothing like what was about to happen in third grade.

In third grade, the students in our district go to a different building. Knowing that, we had thought that it would be best for Alex to be placed in a small, special ed classroom rather than in a mainstream room. The theory was that because there were so many kids, noises, and distractions in a regular classroom, that a quieter, less stimulating classroom would help him feel safe and therefore promote more opportunities for him to grow socially. I had even made sure that the summer before third grade started that Alex and I went to visit the teacher and his new classroom so he could become acquainted with his new surroundings. Let's start school! The first few months were an adjustment, and Alex just didn't seem comfortable there. One particular student had Downs Syndrome, and was non- verbal. He caused such a disruption day to day by running out of the classroom and his constant humming and drooling, that it drove Alex crazy. The teacher finally had to put special handles on the door to keep the kid inside the room. Don't get me wrong, I'm not singling out any one type of disability, it just so happens that the child in question had Downs Syndrome. Another child had multiple behavioral and physical disabilities, and still another one needed the assistance of a wheelchair because he had problems walking.

Work and homework were a joke. Alex would come home with words like "cat," "dog," "pen," and "milk" just to name a few. Math was no better. 1+1, 5-0, 8+2. COME ON. REALLY? Here is a child whose IQ is in the genius range and she is giving him work that he blew through when he was like 2 years old? Note after note, call after call, no response after no response was really getting on my nerves. Alex was obviously bored and acting out because of the lack of structure in the room, the constant distractions and disturbances, and generally the lack of training these people had in dealing with special needs children. The principal was worse. He didn't even care that Alex wasn't learning anything. He kept saying that Alex was the cause of his own abilities to fit in, do his work, etc. What a waste. This guy actually had a doctorate in education. Guess he sent in 5 box tops and they sent it to him in the mail! My frustration got to the point that I had to hire a lawyer that specializes in special ed laws. She was a godsend, and I don't know if I could have made it through without her help. Once the school found out I had hired a lawyer, things changed dramatically. Not for the better, but for the worse. They were now out to get Alex and me for any little thing that happened. Guess they were mad because I actually had decided to fight for what was best for MY child. After that, things were about to get ugly and nasty.

The last straw came at the end of April. I had dropped him off at school in the morning, and went to work. A couple of hours later, I get a phone call saying I have to come and get him. I asked why, but they refused to tell me over the phone. I left work, told my boss I'd be back, and went to the school. As I was entering the building, I saw Alex walking, or should I say limping, down the hall, holding his lunch, with the principal at his side. I also noticed a bruise on his face. I immediately asked the principal what had happened, and he told me that there was an "incident" in the classroom. I figured he meant that another child had hit Alex because of the bruise. Alex is not a fighter, so I knew he wouldn't be the instigator. What the principal told me next absolutely sickened me. It seems as though when Alex was in the "quiet room," which is actually just a partition set up to divide the room and give the kids a few moments to decompress, his teacher went down to get his lunch from the cafeteria(Alex didn't like to eat in the cafeteria because it was much too loud, so they let him eat in the classroom). When she came back, she told him that she was going to leave it on his desk and he could come out whenever he was ready. He acknowledged her and started to come over. When he did, he tripped and knocked the partition over. Two of the aides who were in the classroom thought he did it on purpose. They physically grabbed him and slammed him to the ground. On the way down, he hit his face on a desk, and landed on his hip. He also sustained numerous fingerprint bruises on his arms and wrists from the attack. He began to scream and went into a fight or flight mode. He saw himself in danger and was trying to get out of it. He began swinging to get the aides off of him, and the principal was called to the room. When the principal arrived, he too restrained Alex. Again Alex tried to wriggle out of the danger her was in. He then had a full blown asthma attack and the nurse, principal, and staff REFUSED to give him his inhaler! When I questioned the principal about it, he told me that he didn't feel as though it was necessary for Alex to receive treatment. Seriously, an 8 year old child with Autism has just been physically attacked by two obviously untrained, unqualified aides in a classroom, and you don't see the need for him to breathe?? IT IS ON. Good old "Dr. Clueless" told me to come back later that day for a meeting with him and the CST leader. Before that was going to happen, I had to get Alex to a safe place and make sure there weren't any more serious internal injuries.

I left the building, at the first person I called, right in front of the school, was my lawyer. Needless to say, she was not happy. The next person I called was the pediatrician. He told me to bring Alex right in to be seen. When I got there, he asked what had happened, and Alex, being brutally honest and unable to lie, told him exactly what had happened. He had to excuse himself from the room to regain his composure. When he came back in, he examined Alex and assured him that he wasn't going to hurt him. He also promised him that he wouldn't allow anybody else to hurt him. The pediatrician then told us that there were no broken bones or other life threatening injuries and told us to follow up with him in a couple of weeks.

I went to the meeting later that afternoon, and what happened next is so shocking, that I couldn't believe it. The principal and CST director told me that Alex was being suspended for 10 days do to his aggressive behavior! This is a child who had missed a total of 2 days of school since kindergarten. What a joke. Again, I called my lawyer and she told me to let him serve out the 10 days at home because he would be safer there than in that school building. That was the last time Alex ever stepped foot in that building. I wanted his records. All of them. I wrote a letter to the principal, CST, superintendent, and school board requesting ANY AND ALL records, written or verbal, that pertained to Alex. This included handwritten notes, verbal communication, and e-mails. Guess they thought they could pull the wool over my eyes because when I got the records, there were maybe 50 pages. I knew this wasn't all of them, so I contacted my lawyer. What a surprise, she received a stack with about 500 pages. Funny thing is though, that in the school's haste to get them to us, they gave us some records from another students file. Other records were missing. What a nightmare. I'm happy to report that all those involved with this incident no longer work at the school. They either "retired" or "took employment elsewhere."

As that mess continued, we decided to send Alex to a private school out of district that is for children on the Autism Spectrum and those with behavioral issues. I was really concerned at first, because this was all new to us. My fears were laid to rest however when I met Alex's teacher for the first time. Her name was Ms. Joan. I had filled her in on all the issues we had faced in the previous public school, and she listened intently to what I had to say. She immediately put into place some things that she would try to do to make him feel safe and welcome. One of those things was to institute a no restraint policy unless it was absolutely necessary. The class sizes are small, maybe 5 or 6 kids per room with a teacher and one or two teacher assistants. They are all on the same page, and know what needs to be done for each and every child in the school. This was a refreshing change, because before there was no communication, here there was constant communication. If something needed to be tweaked or fixed, it was. If it worked, it stayed. It wasn't just Ms. Joan that tried, but the entire staff. From the aides to the secretaries, to the special area teachers right on up to the vice principal and principal, Alex was taken in and told that he could do whatever he set as a goal. The staff was also fantastic towards us and kept encouraging us to not give up. It wasn't easy that first year, but with the dedication and help we all received, it was a success. By the end of that 4th grade year, Alex had begun to show signs of his old self. Good signs. He began to come out of his shell a little more and began to smile more. I think at that point, I knew that this was the place he needed to be. I had requested that Alex be placed with Ms. Joan for 5th grade as well. The principal had told me that had already had that idea in mind. In fact, Alex had Ms. Joan for 4th, 5th, 6th, and 7th grade. You would think she would be tired of seeing his and my face for that long right? She absolutely has the best sense of humor, most genuine heart and most loving and caring attitude of not only any teacher I have ever met, but any person I have ever met. I always tell her thank you, but I really cannot thank her enough for taking a scared little boy and creating a fine young man. THANK YOU!! As of this writing, Alex is entering the 8th grade and has a new set of teachers. Keeping my fingers crossed that all will work out. He still has Ms. Joan to go to if the need arises. I made sure of that. To the staff of the school: Thank you too for all you have done to make us all feel welcome and safe.

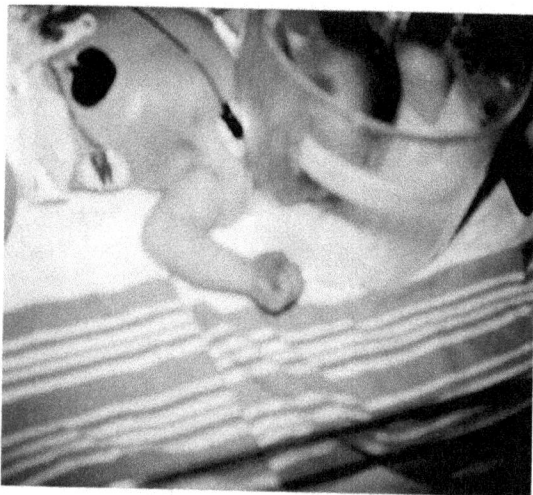

Alex in the incubator

Alexander Keith Smaniotto 6/27/90 6 Lbs. 11 Oz.
19 3/4 Inches

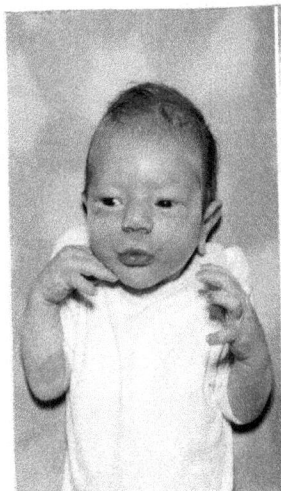

First Halloween October 31, 1998

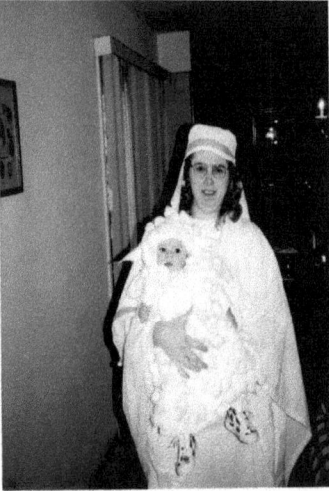

Easter Finery

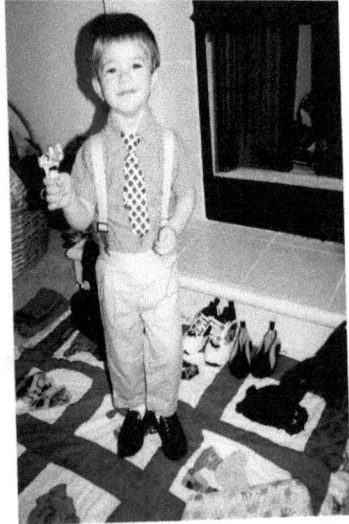

Aren & Daddy looking sharp!

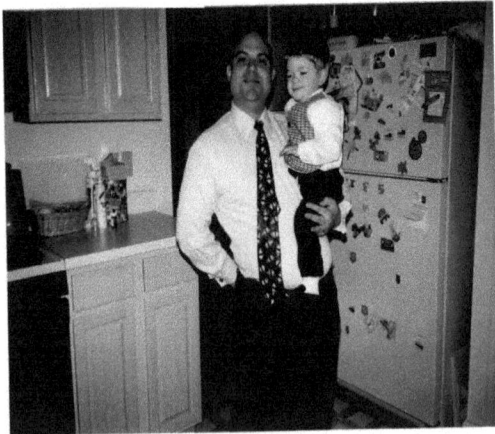

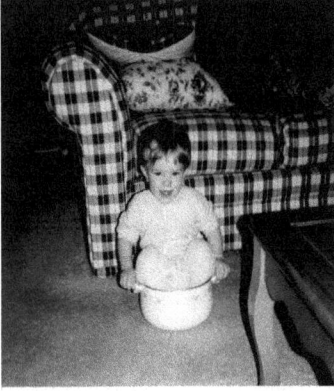

A-nu stew!

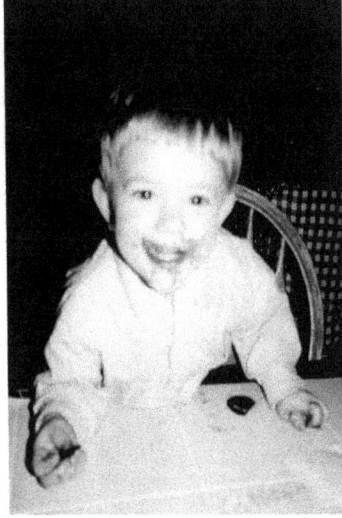

The discovery of Oreos!

Bobbing for mushrooms!

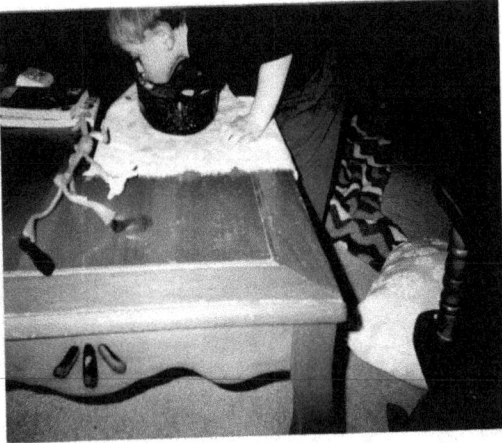

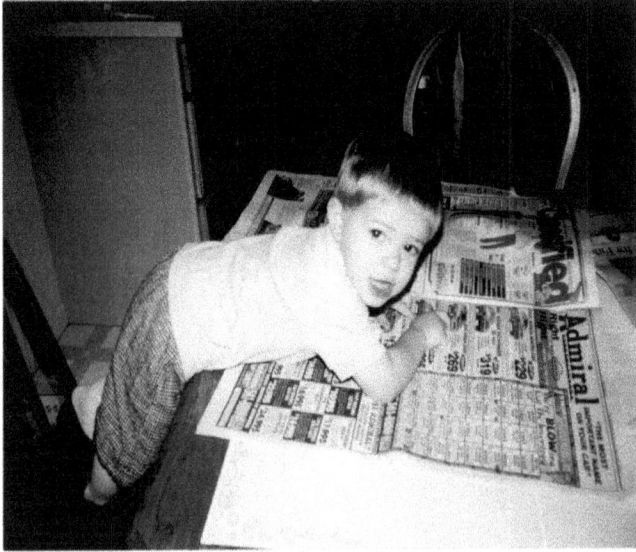

Checking out the Sunday paper to see what car he wants!

Arbu & his cars

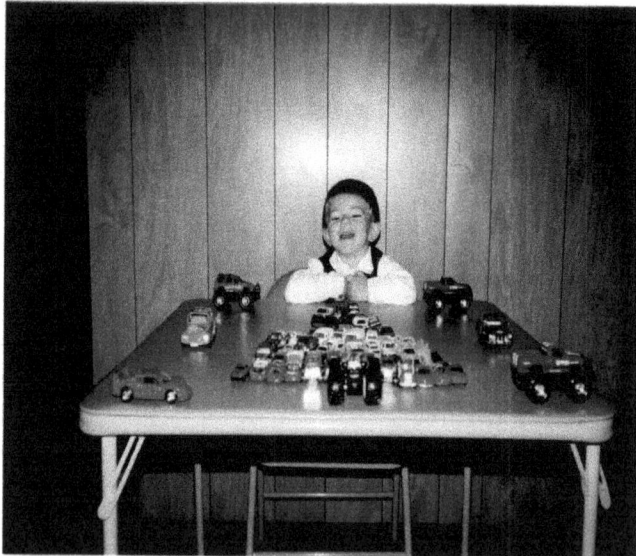

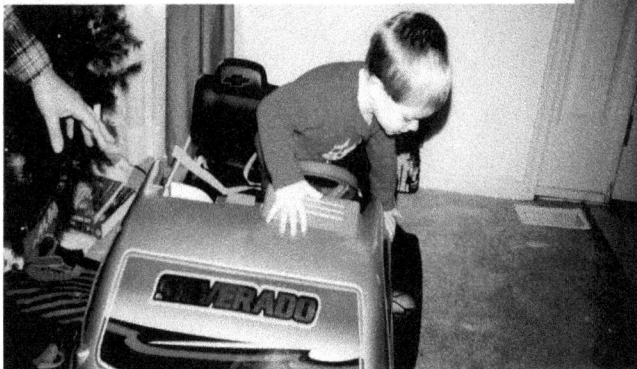

CHEVY SILVERADO!!!!!!!!

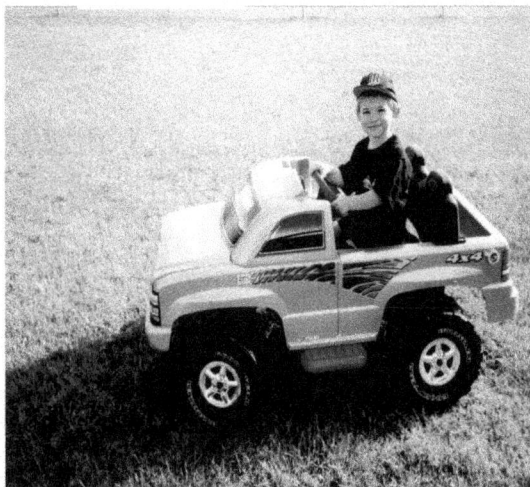

Cruisin' in the Chevy Silverado!

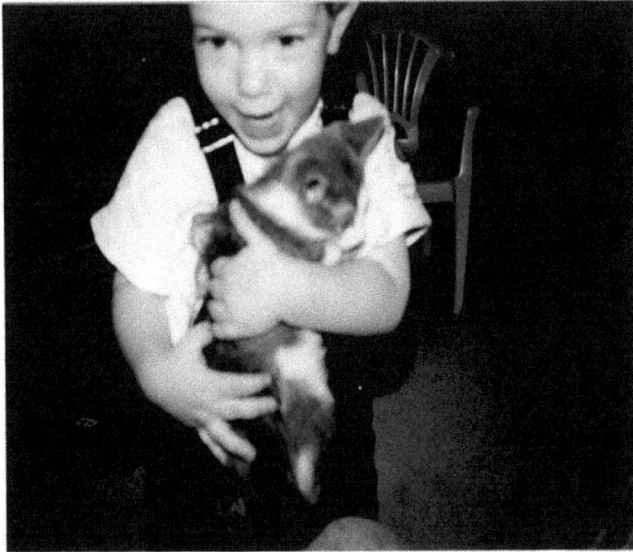

Allen with our cat Tilly

Wiped out!

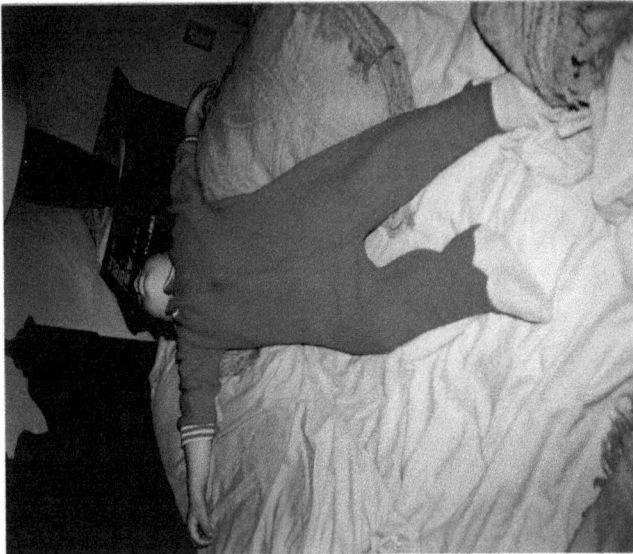

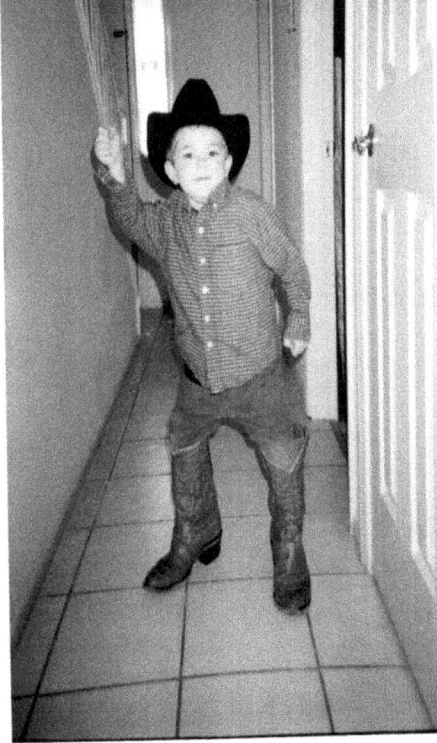
I'm a cowboy!

Grade school photos. Notice he's not smiling in the 3rd grade picture

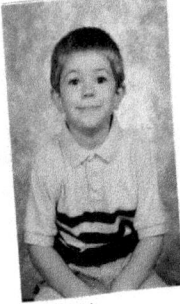

Kindergarten

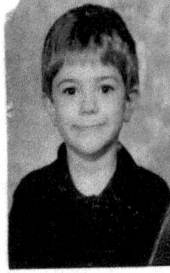

1st grade

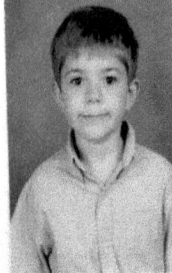

2nd grade

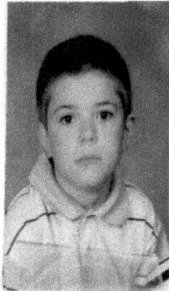

3rd grade. Our nightmare year

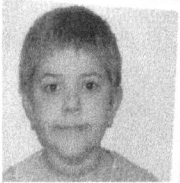

4th grade

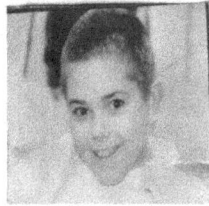

5th grade

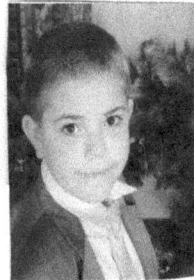

6th grade

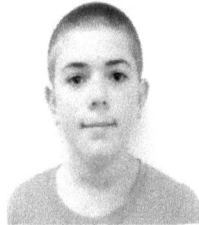

7th grade

7. Tragedy Part 2

As I have mentioned before, my Mom was always there for us. She was a saint. Her smile and sense of humor were unmatched. Her big heart was evident every day of every week of every year. She was the "lunch lady" at the very same school we all had attended, and where Elaine taught. She worked there from the mid 1970's until 2002. In that time, she touched so many lives with her love and generosity. There was more than one time when a child wouldn't have enough money for milk or a lunch, and she would tell her boss that she would pay for it, just let the kid eat. Dropped your burger on the floor? No problem, Mrs. Champion would fix you up. Need help opening your milk or juice, no problem, Mrs. Champion will help you. This next one is one of my favorites because even today kids who needed her help see me and tell me "your Mom peeled my orange for me." Sounds simple, but Mom was always prepared at work. She used to carry an orange peeler in her pocket, just in case someone needed an orange peeled. It also served other purposes that were food related.

Her smile and sense of humor never seemed to leave her, even in the darkest of times. Her laugh was contagious. Never once did I hear her utter "why me?" She just faced whatever challenge was put in front of her and handled it with grace, a smile and a sense of humor. As you may remember, some of those dark times were the death of my sister Elaine, and the near loss of my father. She had faced many deaths and sad times before I was born, but she handled them just as you would expect her to from what I have been told. These things made her stronger, but what was about to happen to her was, I felt, so unfair.

It was mid-1998, and she wasn't feeling well. Alex was just a tiny baby and of course she doted on him. She tried to hide her pain, which she did quite well, I might add. She didn't want to worry any of us, so she kept it to herself. Seems as though she hadn't been feeling well for quite a while, and decided to go to the doctor. He sent her for some tests, and she was just waiting for the results. It was the day before Thanksgiving, and I happened to be at work. When I got a break, I called to see how she was feeling and if she had gotten any news. I could tell she didn't really want to tell me, and her voice was shaking a little bit. "Breast cancer." I was heartbroken once again. I kept thinking "not again." I was not ready to face the possibility that I could now lose my Mom to this terrible disease too. She told the doctor that she had to wait until after the holidays to get treatment because she didn't want to ruin Christmas for her children and grandchildren. Shortly thereafter, she had a mastectomy. She began getting chemotherapy and of course it had the usual side effects. She had nausea, and was in some considerable pain, but she didn't want anyone to worry about her. That was just her style. When she started losing her hair, she teased Keith that now they looked alike. When Keith and I started dating and then got married, she used to tease us and say "too bad you had to get a bald headed one!" You may have guessed from this statement that Keith is bald. She continued to work as much as she could, but sometimes she just couldn't. I know that bothered her because she loved her job and she loved the kids. She finished her treatments, and things were looking up. She had stayed strong, kept her sense of humor and her smile, and most importantly, she never gave up. She went for regular checkups, and at one point was declared cancer free. We were so happy! That joy didn't last long though because a couple of years later it returned. This time, it had turned into breast, ovarian and lung cancer. Pretty grim prognosis, but again, she stayed strong and used that smile and humor to face it head on. She was about to turn 70, so my siblings and I, knowing that this was probably the last chance we would get to celebrate with her, decided to throw her a surprise 70th birthday party. We managed to get almost every member of our family, including her siblings and their children, grandchildren, and their spouses together in one place. That place was my house. She was surprised! Mission accomplished. We all checked on her frequently, almost daily if we could, to see if she needed anything and see how she was feeling. She would tell us that she was ok, but we could tell that she was getting tired and weak. In early June of 2002, she wasn't feeling well and was having breathing difficulties, so she was hospitalized. The covering oncologist kept telling her "it's the disease and nothing else." She knew her body and knew that it was "something else." She never asked any of us for help, but one day the phone rang and it was her. She said "get me out of here before they kill me." That's all it took. I called Mart, and we both went to work. We had to have called thirty or forty doctors and hospitals looking for someone to take her case. Finally, we found one. It was a hospital in Philadelphia. They set everything up and had a transport ambulance come down here and get her. Within minutes of her arrival, she had numerous doctors and residents looking over her case. When we got there, the head oncologist said to us "you know she has pneumonia, right?" Mom was right and the local oncologist was wrong. Now the thing was can they do anything about it? She was treated with IV antibiotics, and about a week and a half later she was ready to be sent home. The doctor in Philadelphia agreed to allow her to come back home here for her radiation and chemotherapy, because Mom just didn't think she could stand the ride 5 days a week to get radiation up in the city.

The decision had already been made by us that when she was released, she would not be going back to her house. She would come to live with one of us. We gave her the choice, and she picked my house since it was the biggest and she figured it would be a little less crowded since it was just 3 of us compared to 5 at Mart's.

As the day arrived for her to come home, it was a little hectic, to say the least. I couldn't get off of work to be there when she got home, which really upset me, but there was nothing I could do about it. My aunt went to the house to sign for the hospital bed. Furniture needed to be moved to get a space ready downstairs for her, and we had to figure out how she was going to walk up the short set of steps at my front door. Everything fell into place. I got done work and came home. I got Mom settled for the night and gave her a baby monitor we used for Alex, and headed to bed. She had a rough first night, but we tried our best. She didn't want to bother me, so she just tried to do things herself. I told her all she had to do was call upstairs by speaking in to the monitor, but again, she didn't want to bother us. She started radiation on that Monday and went daily for treatments. She was able to walk for about the first week or so, but then it became really difficult for her, so we had a wheelchair brought in. After her treatment on Thursday, August 8, she came home and was excited. I asked her what was going on, and she told me that for the first time in a long time she could breathe. I was really happy and thought that maybe that was just what she needed. Mart brought her kids up that day too, and things seemed to be looking up. The next morning, Keith had gone downstairs and was getting ready to go to work. He talked to her and then left. About half an hour later, I went down and she was sitting in the chair. She looked pale and was saying things that didn't make sense. I asked her if she was alright, and she said she had been calling for help for hours. I knew Keith had just recently left, and I called him at work to ask him about it. He said they had a perfectly normal conversation and he told her he was leaving for work. She said ok and she'd see him later. I told him he had to come home. NOW. I hung up the phone and called her hospice worker. She came over a few minutes after my Dad got there. I had asked Holly (remember her) the day before if she could watch Mom on Friday so I could run some errands. She said yes. When the hospice worker got there, she pulled Dad and I aside and said "she's actively dying right now." We were stunned. At this point, Holly had just gotten there, I believe, and we told her what was happening. I also had to track down Mart, Vernon and John. Alex was still upstairs, and I was worried about him. I called my aunt and told her what was going on. Without hesitation, she came to my house and took Alex with her back to her house. She was in the midst of moving, so it wasn't like she needed any extra stress either, but she and I both knew that he would be better off there than here. Before Alex left, I made sure he hugged Mom and told her that he loved her. She did the same. It was the last time they would see each other. I was able to track down Mart, but I was having real difficulties finding Vernon and John. I called my work and just lost it on the phone when I told my boss what was going on. She offered to call around and try to find Vernon for me. I finally got in touch with him and told him to come up right now. He was engaged at the time, and his wedding was only a few months away (He would become a step-dad to Jen's teenaged daughter Shelby, even though he never had kids of his own). He began thinking about how he would be the only one of her children that she wouldn't see get married. I felt really bad for him. He and his fiancée came up, and he had called his best friend too. The friend came up and let Mom know he was there. We had everyone who showed up that day do the same so that Mom would know how much she was loved. Joanne works at the hospital, so I had called there looking for her to get in touch with John. The nurse there said Joanne wasn't working, but she would find her. Within a few minutes, John called and was on his way up. He had been getting ready to go camping (I think) with his church group and was packing up the gear which is why he didn't answer when I called. I called my best friend Jane, and she came right away. Ironically, 6 weeks to the day that my Mom died, her Mom died of cancer too. The next step was to get in touch with Mom's siblings. One by one we reached them, and they all made their way down to my house. We weren't able to reach her younger brother (who has the same birth date as her) in time. He and his wife had been away for the day so they weren't there when she died. All of her other brothers and sisters made it though. With her family surrounding her, Mom fought and fought until the very end. A couple of times Mart took her hand and told her to pass over and be with Elaine and her own sister Ethel who had died of cancer too. She wasn't ready to go. Finally, at around 8 PM that evening, with Vernon and Mart holding her hands and my Dad and myself rubbing her back, she passed away. It was a devastating blow to the entire family. Things would never be the same again.

As we planned yet another funeral, the outpouring of love and support from the community, family and friends continued to overwhelm us. This woman who touched so many lives would be remembered for her kindness, her smile, and her sense of humor. As the viewing and funeral took place, it was very evident just how much Mom was loved by everyone who knew her. The line stretched for what seemed like an eternity, and every person there spoke of her love of family, love of life, and her strength and smile in times of adversity.

I had written a eulogy that I wanted to read, but when I got up there I joked that I couldn't read it and just threw the paper away. I spoke from the heart, and I believe that has to have been one of the toughest things I had ever done in my life. I hope if Mom was watching from above, that she liked it and that I made her proud. After all, I learned from the best. It was very evident that Mom was there with us all when different people spoke during the service. My aunt, she and her husband were the ones that just missed being there when Mom passed, got up and started laughing because she realized she had two different color shoes on. She quipped that she had another pair at home just like them! Everybody laughed. Mom would have too. As the service drew to a close, it was time to face the fact that my Mom, who had been there through thick and thin, good and bad, laughter and tears, was gone. Again, no goodbyes, just see you later. Godspeed Mom and Elaine, I will see you both again someday. I can hear her laughter and see her smiling face to this day. She taught me alot, and that has come in handy for what I am about to tell you now. Thank you Mom.

Mom & Dad on their wedding day

Mom & Dad before her illness

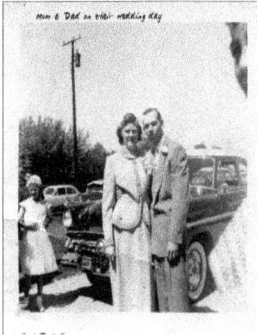

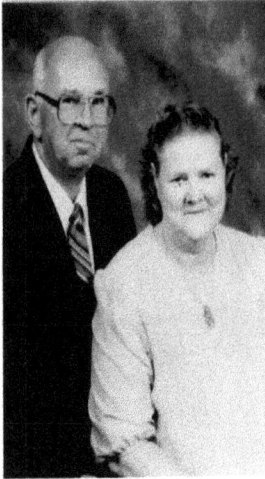

Mom & Dad after her illness

Still smiling

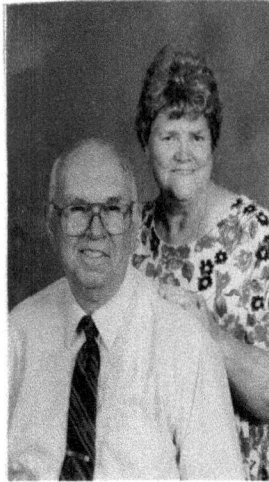

Last family photo before Elaine died

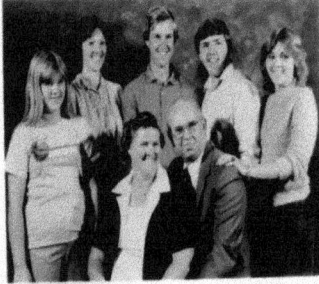

Family photo. Vernon, Mart's husband Don, Mart, Me, Mom
& Dad. John wasn't able to make it.

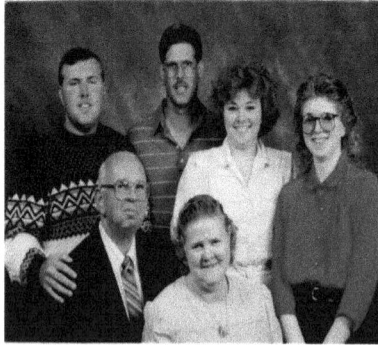

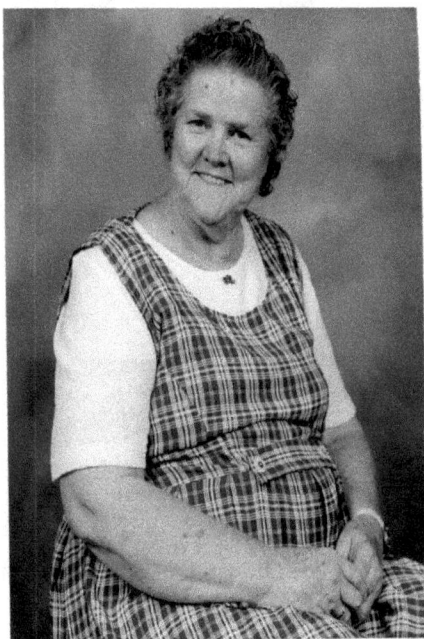
Mom smiling as always

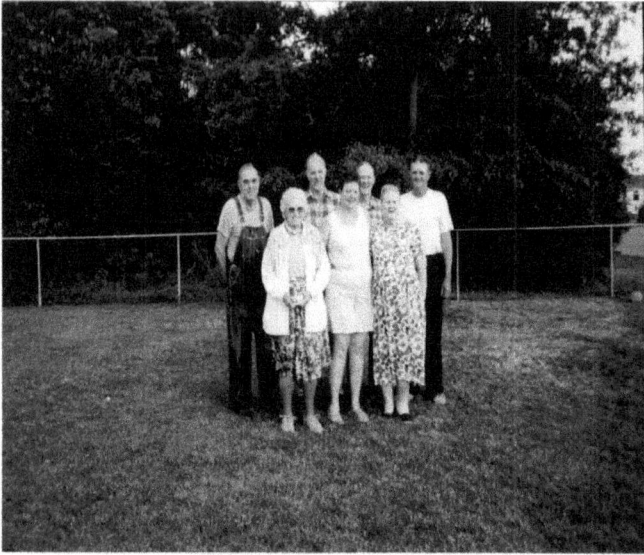

Mom with her siblings at her 70th birthday party. Leon, Willis, Jake, Herbie, Mom, Annamae, & Charlotte.

The ENTIRE Errickson Clan at Mom's 70th birthday party

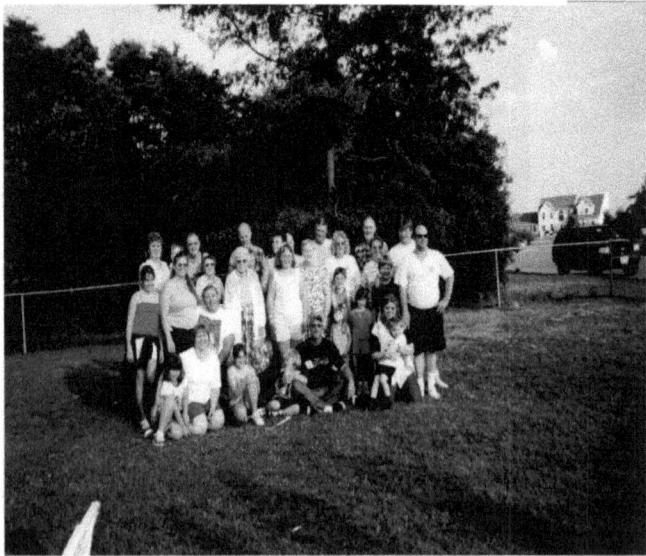

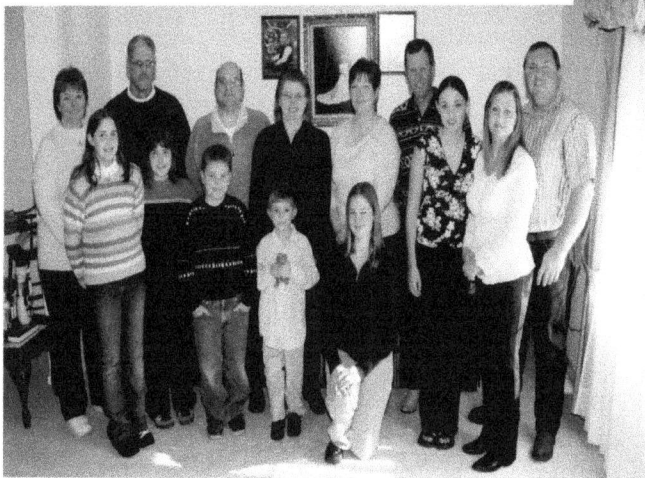

The entire Champion Clan. Mart, Don, Keith, Me, Joanne, John, Shelby, Jen, Vernon, Anna, Alex, JJ, Fran & Steph. This was a photo for Dad's 75th birthday

8. The True Test has Begun

You got all that, right? Good because this is where all the fun really begins! We have a saying in our family that nothing good ever comes out of an even numbered year. Ever since 1988 when Elaine died, it seems that all the bad things happen in even numbered years. Dad's accident 1990, Keith and I get married 1996 (haha), Mom died 2002. I'm now entering 2008, so this can't be good.

There is a saying that God only gives you what you can handle. He must think I can handle a lot. I mean A LOT. This chapter is about the real reason I wrote this book, but I felt I needed to give you some background on what I have dealt with in my life. I believe that those events were the precursor to my greatest challenge yet, so here we go.

As I said, my journey begins on May 29, 2008 or shortly before. Back in 2004, I suffered a miscarriage and no one knew why. I went to a fertility specialist to figure out why. He did some tests and blood work and when they came back, I was told there seemed to be nothing out of the ordinary. We just chalked it up to bad luck. Years later it would all make sense. You know the saying "if I knew then what I know now?" Well, that certainly applies here. The first sign that something was really wrong was on November 9, 2007. I visited my family doctor because I was having difficulty breathing. She sent me for a chest x-ray just to make sure nothing was going on in there. Of course it was a Friday afternoon, so I wouldn't have any results until at least Monday or Tuesday. She told me that if I had any problems over the weekend, go to the emergency room. By the time Saturday morning rolled around, I really couldn't breathe. I went to the emergency room, and the doctor ordered blood work and a CT scan to see what was going on. When the results came back, the CT scan didn't really show anything abnormal. When the blood work came back, it showed that something called D-Dimer was elevated to 1100. A normal D-Dimer is well below 500. This particular test detects the presence of a clot somewhere in the body. The ER doctor told me that sometimes the D-Dimer test comes back elevated if the person is under a lot of stress. We passed it off as that, and he sent me home. He said to follow up with my family doctor on Monday and tell her what had happened. I did, and the doctor agreed that it was probably just stress related. We left it at that. In the weeks following that event, I still had no energy, couldn't multitask like I was used to, found simple things difficult to do, and was exhausted. I don't mean tired, I mean exhausted. I was working, taking care of Alex, who you now know has his own issues, and was preparing for the upcoming Thanksgiving and Christmas holidays. I muddled through it, and after Christmas, I let out a big sigh of relief that it was finally over. That didn't last long. On December 27, I woke up around midnight and was just really, really weak, almost paralyzed. I felt horrible. I woke Keith up and told him to call the ambulance. By the time they arrived, I was so weak, my speech was slurred,

I had a massive headache, and I couldn't see out of my right eye. They took one look at me and told Keith that they were sure I had had a stroke. On the way to the hospital, they started an IV, hooked me up to a monitor, and tried to ask me questions which I just couldn't answer because I couldn't get the words from my brain to my mouth. We finally arrived at the ER, and the medics told the doctor what the situation was. They told him that they were sure that I had a stroke. He walked over, glanced at me, told the medics "No she didn't, it's a migraine." They argued with each other for several minutes while I lay there waiting for someone to help me. The doctor told them that I didn't fit the profile to have a stroke at my age because I didn't smoke, drink, or have a family history of stroke. Finally, the doctor came over and said that they were going to give me some medication in the IV for my "migraine." The nurse came in and gave me something, and that was the last time I saw any medical staff for 3 hours. The doctor came back and told me they were sending me home now. I just looked at him like he was crazy. I still couldn't see, I was really weak, and was having trouble speaking. They didn't even do any blood work, CT scan or actual physical exam. Remember, the doctor just came in and glanced at me. He didn't even do the follow the light with your eyes exam. At that point, I remember thinking, that if I didn't leave, they were going to kill me because it was obvious that they didn't believe me and just didn't care. I called Keith and told him to come get me before they did kill me.

Over the next couple of weeks, I got progressively worse. I was nowhere near my former self, and no one could figure out what was wrong with me. All I knew was that there was something drastically wrong with my body, and no one seemed to believe me. I was still having very limited vision in my right eye, and as luck would have it, I was due for an appointment at my eye doctor. I told him the issues I was having, and when he did the eye exam he said that it looked like a blood clot had passed through my eye and may have injured my optic nerve. Now I was really worried. I couldn't figure out why none of the other doctors had thought of this especially when the D-Dimer came back so high. I guess they figured that if there wasn't an active clot in my chest or lungs, then it must have been a false positive. I happen to have a neighbor who is a semi-retired doctor. He knew I was having trouble and checked up on me pretty regularly to see if there was any change. When I told him about this new finding, he suggested that I see a neurologist. Just so happens that he had helped train one of the top neurologists in the area when he was still an intern. I called the neurologist right away, but had difficulty getting through. I finally got an appointment, but they told me that they were booked until the middle of July. It was only February at that point, so I figured I would just have to tough it out until then and hope for the best. After all, I had been sick this long, what would a few more months of waiting hurt, right? When I told my neighbor about the wait, he called the office for me himself. He was able to get me in at the end of May, but at least it was better than July. They told me to get my hands on any and all records that I could from the past months. I did, and finally the day came for me to see him. I thought to myself that this hour and a half drive in both directions better be worth it and not come up as another dead end.

May 27, 2008 was the day that eventually would end up becoming the beginning of a life long journey. I didn't know it at the time, but it was going to get worse before it got better. I saw the doctor and he did the basic overview exam in the office. He performed a couple of tests that day too, and told me to follow up with him in about two weeks to go over the test results and the previous months paperwork. I made the appointment, but never got that far.

On May 29, I was at work and still not feeling well. One of the pharmacists looked over at me and asked if I was alright. Just as she said that, I got this overwhelming feeling of sickness and down I went. Guess what? I had just had a stroke. She wanted to call the ambulance, but I told her no because I knew that they would take me to the same hospital that just a few months before had not believed me when I was there. I had her call my neurologist instead. When they got ahold of him, he wanted to see me right away. I left work and somehow managed to get to his office. When he had looked at the previous blood work and CT scan, he found something that the ER doctor had missed. A tiny blood clot in my lung. He told me in no certain terms that I was lucky to be alive and that it was so scary to him that they missed something that important. He told me that I had indeed had a stroke as far back as that November 2007 date. Since there was no documentation at all for the December visit, he couldn't prove it, but it was a pretty much a given at that point. I have said I will never go back to that ER again if something happens. I will go in the Northerly direction, not Southbound.

Here are just a couple of interesting or ironic facts:

70 age that my Mom died

-32 age that Elaine died

=38 the age that I finally got diagnosed with my illnesses

HMM.

The next few weeks and months were unbelievable. My head still spins when I think of everything that happened so quickly after waiting so long for an answer. Once the neurologist got the results, he began ordering test after test to try and figure out what was going on. Along with having blood work done quite frequently, he sent me for such tests as ECG, TEE, MRI, MRV, a carotid ultrasound and other miscellaneous things. I had never heard of some of the tests he ordered, but I figured it would be worth it to find out what was wrong with me. I thought that there was finally a doctor who took the time to listen to me and make me feel like he believed me and that these problems weren't in my head.

As the results came trickling in, he became concerned and told me he wanted me to see a cardiologist. He recommended one from the same hospital he works at, so I took his advice and made an appointment. Things did not look good. On July 3, 2008, I went to see the cardiologist. She did an EKG in the office, and said to me "when did you have your heart attack?" I said "not heart attack, stroke." She said, " heart attack AND stroke." Apparently, I had a silent heart attack and didn't even know it. Here I am, 38 years old, and have just been told that in the past few months I have had not one, but two catastrophic medical events. She immediately ordered a stress test and pulmonary function tests to see what kind of damage had already been done. Needless to say, neither of the tests went well. I had to wear a heart monitor for 21 days, and then another one right after that for 1 day. These monitors recorded any abnormalities that the heart may have or develop. She ordered blood work too because there was something in the previous ones that didn't sit well with her. When those results came back, she told me I needed to see a hematologist. I asked her if I could go local on this one because by now the 3 hour round trip drives were taking a toll on me. I couldn't imagine having to make another weekly trip up there to see another specialist. The cardiologist agreed, and I chose a hematologist who has the reputation of being one of the top ones locally in her field. I also picked her because she had treated my Mom and was so kind and caring towards her. Before I went for my actual appointment though I wanted to drop off my tests and blood work so she could look over it before I first saw her. On the day I did that, she happened to be at the desk and saw me come in. She recognized me and said "What are you doing in my office. You don't have cancer do you?" I told her that I was having blood issues, and she breathed a sigh of relief. On July 10, I got in to see her. She had looked over the previous months nightmare, and ordered a ton, and I mean a ton, of blood work of her own. She wanted me to get a CT scan of my chest and abdomen while we were waiting for the results of the blood work. I also was still having tests ordered by the neurologist and cardiologist, so I was being pulled in a hundred different directions at once. Almost lost in this is the fact that I had to see an ear nose and throat specialist because during the previous brain MRI, it had been discovered that I had a nasal polyp that was going to need to be operated on. That seemed like the least of my worries at that point, but it actually was pretty significant later. By this point, I was just plain exhausted. Finally after a couple of weeks the blood work came back. I went to the hematologist's office on July 29, and we went through the results bit by bit. She eliminated everything that I didn't have, which was good, but then she told me that I had tested positive for something called Antiphospholipid Syndrome (APS). I had no idea what that was, and I knew I couldn't say it! Can you repeat that? Maybe write it down? She explained to me that APS is a rare, incurable autoimmune/blood clotting disorder where the body recognizes blood or cell membranes as a foreign substance and develops antibodies against them. If left untreated, it can cause strokes, heart attacks, miscarriages and a host of other problems. It usually strikes women who are in their 30's and 40's, although it can happen to those younger or older, and rarely men get it. Everything started to fall into place now. The stroke, the heart attacks, the constant fatigue, the memory loss, the inability to do the things I used to be able to do and the miscarriages I suffered in 2004 (evidently, my APS levels were high back then, but no one bothered to tell me that) all had a cause now. I felt like finally someone was going to help me get through this. I asked her what the next step was since she had told me there is no cure. She said that I would have to take anticoagulants for the rest of my life to keep my blood in check. Having worked in the pharmacy for almost 20 years at that point, I was hesitant at first about taking them. Then I realized, if I don't do this, I WILL die. I wouldn't get to see Alex grow up and I didn't want Alex to grow up without a Mom. At that point, it was time to fight. I knew my enemy, and I was ready to take it down! She started me on a regimen of both injectable and oral medications to help bring the levels down to a more acceptable range. For the first month or so, I saw her 2 or 3 times per week. These visits were to draw blood and check the levels. If the anticoagulants needed to be adjusted, that is how we would know. Believe me, those doses changed often! While we were in this trial and error period, she said that because of my family history of breast cancer, it might not be a bad idea to get tested for the breast cancer gene. I said sure, why not. My cousin had been diagnosed with breast cancer a few years before, and she had the test done. If you remember, her Mom, my aunt, was the one that died in the 1960's from it. We used her test results to determine if there was indeed a family link to this deadly disease. On September 23, I got a phone call from the hematologist's office asking me to come in to speak with the doctor. It was pretty obvious what the result was going to be. I had tested positive for BRCA2, breast and ovarian cancer mutations. Because my results matched genetically with my cousin's, it was determined that we had a family mutation. There is a very high probability that my Mom, Elaine and my aunt all had the defective gene. There were several options presented to me about how to treat it. I could have mammograms twice a year, just monitor it and see what would happen, or I could eliminate the threat all together by having a prophylactic hysterectomy and double mastectomy. The combination of me having the APS and BRCA2 was not a good one. I was now at a higher risk of developing breast and or ovarian cancer in the future. I was not willing to take that risk. The option I picked for myself was a no brainer. Hysterectomy and double mastectomy. People questioned me as to why I would "mutilate" my body by having this done. I really kind of resented them asking me that. It is my body, and I am doing what I need to do to survive and see Alex grow up. Again the thought of not being here to see Alex grow up was too much for me to bear. I HAVE to be here for him. People also asked me what Keith thought about the whole thing. I told them that he knew that the door was always open for him to get out if he couldn't handle it. I again explained to those people that it was my body and only I had the right to make a decision about what needed to be done. For some strange reason, Keith stayed!

An ultrasound was ordered just to make sure that there were no problems developing, and thankfully, there weren't. I made an appointment with my gynecologist because he would be the one doing the hysterectomy. We spoke, and he agreed that if he were in my shoes he would do the same thing. Since it was now early October, I knew that I would have to wait until after the holidays to have it done. I couldn't be out of commission for Christmas, because Alex was only 10 at the time. It wouldn't have been fair to ruin his Christmas.

In the meantime, I needed to get the polyp removed. I started with the least invasive procedure first to see how well I would be able to tolerate surgery with my newly diagnosed condition. Because of the APS, and the increase risk of bleeding from surgery, I had to be off of the anticoagulants so that my blood would thicken up. It sounds like an oxymoron because the idea is to get my blood thinner so that I won't get a clot, but for surgery, they don't want it too thin because then I could bleed to death. Catch 22. I was a little nervous about it, but all the doctors closely monitored me before, during and after the surgery. On October 28, I was wheeled into surgery to have the polyp removed. It turns out that it was a good thing I had it done because the polyp was blocking about 70% to 80% of my nasal passage. That was part of the reason I was having such difficulty breathing. Wouldn't you know it, on October 29, my beloved Philadelphia Phillies won their first World Series in 28 years and I couldn't even jump up and down and cheer! I had to cheer them on gently from the couch! I guess that was a small price to pay to be able to breathe somewhat normally again.

Thanksgiving and Christmas came, and I tried to keep things as normal as possible for Alex. I knew that in a few short days that my dream of ever having another child would come to an end. I grieved a little, but then I looked at the child I already had and thought to myself that I was the luckiest Mom around. Alex is special and I thought how wonderful it was that God had chosen me to be that special child's mother. Even though he was only 10 at the time, he was wise beyond his years. We didn't try to hide anything from him and I answered his questions about my conditions the best way that I could. I could tell he was very scared, but at the same time I knew that as long as he knew what was happening, he would be able to prepare for what was going to happen.

On December 29, 2008, I was once again wheeled in to surgery. This time, it was for the hysterectomy. To say that I wasn't my normal, cheery, upbeat self after I came out of surgery is an understatement! I had never been in so much pain in my life. As I had said before, I'm not a person who takes medication for every little thing, so when I was offered narcotics through my IV, I declined. The nurse could see how much pain I was in and said take the pain medication, because I really needed it. I agreed, but it didn't even begin to numb the pain. What happened next was probably my most awful reaction to the pain. When the doctor came in to check on me, he had brought an intern with him. He began to remove the bandage to show her the incision. As he was doing that, it hurt REALLY badly, so I kicked him in the groin! I don't know if he remembers that, but I sure do. I felt really bad, and that was not one of my finest moments. From that point on, when he would come in to check on me, he would stand back from the bed and ask me how I was feeling. At that point, his partner came in to check on me too. He could see that the IV medication was not even touching the pain, so he told the nurse to discontinue the IV and give me oral pain medication from now on. They were giving me narcotic pain relievers two at a time to help, and believe me, they knocked me out, which was a good thing. A few days after the surgery, I was finally starting to feel a little better. My hematologist came in and said that I was scaring her because she had never seen me be anything other than strong and upbeat. She said that it was out of character for me, but that she knew this was going to be a hard thing for me to do. I understood what she meant because she and I have a good relationship. On January 1, 2009, I was discharged. When I got home, Alex had drawn some pictures that said "Yeah, Mommy's home." I thought that was the sweetest thing he could have done, and once again he had amazed me with his strength and compassion. I knew then that he would be ok with what was happening.

Let's put 2008 in perspective. Between May 27th and December 31, I had a stroke, a heart attack, got diagnosed with a rare, incurable autoimmune/ blood clotting disease, tested positive for BRCA2 breast and ovarian cancer mutated gene, had surgery to remove a polyp that was blocking most of my nasal passage, and finally, had a hysterectomy. I went to a total of 7 different doctors, had 14 tests done, 2 surgeries and had gone to those doctors a total of 53 times all in a little over 6 months! Whew! What would 2009 have in store? We were about to find out.

Before I continue, let me take a minute to recognize my family, my friends and my church members for supporting me. My family and friends were always there for me, and I knew that. What I found out however, was that my church family would be there for me not only spiritually, but for the everyday things you don't normally think about. The women of the church made sure that we were well fed. One woman even came to clean the house for me several times, and boy was that a huge help. To all of you, a heartfelt and big thank you.

Of course the year started off with me home recovering from the hysterectomy. As I was healing from that, I prepared for the next round of surgery. Before that would happen though, I had already had 9 doctors appointments, one of which was a visit to the emergency room because I had an allergic reaction to a medication I was given.

Friday, February 13, 2009 was a bitterly cold day. I was scheduled to have the mastectomy first thing in the morning, Once again, I was wheeled into the operating room and the surgery was done. Before I knew it, I was in the recovery room being told that all went well. I was still pretty out of it, but at least it didn't hurt as much as the hysterectomy. I was supposed to be kept overnight and come home the next morning, but when the lab drew my blood, it was way too thick for the doctor to allow me to go home. Happy Valentine's Day! Enjoy your stay. I was very disappointed that I wasn't going home, but it was for the best. At that point, I was still wrapped with a heavy duty bandage with drains coming from either side. The drains were put in to help the excess blood and fluid come out of my system. Each time the drains were emptied, the amount of blood in them needed to be measured. I was sent home on Sunday, February 15th. I was told that it was ok to shower, so that was one of the first things I did. I took the bandage off, and the first thing that happened was the drains dropped. They felt like they were pulling my insides out which made sense since they were sewn inside my chest cavity. This was also the first time I would get a look at my new body. I really wasn't prepared for what I was about to see. With the bandage removed, I got a glimpse of my now flat chest. It was being held together with at least 50 staples. I thought I was going to pass out. For the first time since this whole ordeal started, I shed some tears. I think reality had finally started to settle in. Keith, in his usual open mouth insert foot way, said to me "oh, you are finally showing some emotion about the whole thing." Not the smartest thing to say to me at that point. If I had had the strength or energy at that point, Keith would have been missing a certain body part! The shower felt really good because the flow of the water was very soothing. It was a bit difficult though because every time I tried to wash my back or feet, the drains would pull and hurt like heck. As the week progressed, I got a little stronger. The drains and staples were going to be removed, and I couldn't wait. I was tired of bumping them every time I moved. Removing the staples proved the easiest part of the process. They didn't hurt as much as I had expected. The drains on the other hand, were another story. Because they were actually sewn inside my chest, they had started to grow attached to my skin. Removing them proved a little more difficult. The tubes that the drain bulbs were attached to were a few feet long. Add that to the ingrown stitches and you get a very uncomfortable feeling. Once the stitches were removed, and the tugging of the drain tubes began, I almost hit the ceiling thinking "oh my gosh, was this worth it?" It was. By the way, I joked that getting my breasts removed was the easiest 4 pounds I had ever lost! Who knew they were that big, right? LOL! I chose not to do reconstructive surgery, because of a couple of things. First, it would mean me having to go under the knife again for many more hours and that would be dangerous. Secondly, I am not a vain person, and it is more important to me what is on the inside, not what someone looks like on the outside. I figured that this was what God wanted for me, and those who truly know me know exactly how I feel. I still get some stares to this day when I go out and people realize that I have a flat chest. I don't feel the need to explain myself unless I am asked about it. I hold my head high and know that I am lucky to be alive. Again, outward appearances are not the true measure of a person. What is inside is more important.

Once I had started to heal, the doctor thought that physical therapy may help strengthen my upper body and help me regain some of the strength lost from the stroke. There was little improvement, so I stopped doing it.

It was now April, and I had already logged 18 more appointments and many more miles. My neurologist wanted me to have something called a neuro-psych test. Basically it is a very long involved test where they give you hands on things to do along with written items to test your cognitive abilities. It lasted about 8 hours. I knew I was in trouble when the first question they asked me was "what's in water?" I had no clue what they meant. I thought they meant something like the chemicals or flavorings. For the record, the correct answer is Hydrogen and Oxygen-H2O. Duh! I knew for the first time that I was in big trouble neurologically and that my mind was no longer going to be able to think in the way in which I had been able to before. After that test, I still had to drive home. Eight hours of testing and 3 hours round trip driving left me totally exhausted at that point. It's ironic that even today with all my memory issues, certain things stand out. I remember that testing day because it happened to have been done on the same day that Phillies great Harry Kalas died. Weird, another Phillies connection. The test results came back a few weeks later, and big surprise here, I failed the test. There was now a documented, proven brain deficit.

April and May brought 8 more appointments and 1 new doctor. I was still having the breathing difficulties, so off to a new pulmonologist I go. He ordered more pulmonary function tests and something called a blood gases test. If you've never had the pleasure of having blood gases drawn, let me enlighten you about it. They stick a needle in the artery in your wrist, wiggle it around a bit, and draw out the arterial gases. It's not like when the stick your vein to draw blood, that I've since grown used to. It hurts-alot! I still cringe when I think of that one. When the tests come back, they find out that I have very mild asthma. Ok, I can deal with that. They try a ton of different medications, most of which I am allergic to, so we just let it ride and hope that I don't need an inhaler or anything to treat it. The pulmonologist now wants me to have a sleep study. Why on earth they call it a sleep study, I'll never know. You don't actually get any sleep while hooked up to the tons of electrodes and wires. The test comes back that I have mild sleep apnea, so the doc wants to do another one to confirm it and set me up with a CPAP machine. I do the tests and get a CPAP machine. It doesn't help at all, so the machine is discontinued.

As June comes in, my neurologist wants me to have something called a Digi-trace done because I have developed this severe, uncontrollable twitching in my feet and legs at night. It doesn't hurt while it's happening, but by the time morning rolls around, I can just barely walk. I'll describe it like this. My feet and ankles actually feel like they disconnect from my legs and they spin, uncontrollably like a helicopter. The episodes last anywhere from a few seconds to sometimes an hour or more. There is nothing I can do to stop them from doing it, so I just have to ride it out. The test consists of putting electrodes all over your head and wrapping it up so you look like a giant cotton swab. Don't worry though, because you also get a little stretchy type of material to put on over it to keep everything in place. The monitor is one that you carry with you all day, and there is a special monitor that records video of you at night so they can get not only a neurological reading, but a video image too. This goes on for 48 hours. Boy, hope that's not going to end up on You Tube! The tests come back as inconclusive, so now on to the next step.

Going to the hematologist every week is starting to get tiresome, since all they do is take a tube of blood, check it and adjust the dosage of my medication if need be. Sometimes I have to sit there for more than an hour just to have that 2 minute blood work done. The doctor orders me a home INR monitor that allows me to check my blood at home once a week and report in to her. This way, I only have to see her once a month. She also says that it's time for me to get a DEXA scan which measures bone density. It shows some osteopenia, a precursor to osteoporosis, so she puts me on calcium and Vitamin D to stave off any more damage.

As the year progresses, I get more and more symptoms and side effects from the APS. I get more fatigued (not normal fatigue, but literally cannot get off the couch fatigue), start having more severe memory loss, more twitching, and more weakness. I am growing frustrated because I have never not been able to do the things that I wanted or needed to do. I have always been very active, can multi task with the best of them, keep working long hours and other day to day mundane things. That has now been taken away from me, and I don't know how to react, and I know I don't like it. I never before had to stop what I was doing to take a nap or catch my breath. I wonder if my life will ever be the way it was before. I soon realize that it won't. My state disability benefits are long gone, and since it's been over a year that I've been out of work, I can now apply for Social Security Disability benefits. Easier said than done. That will be explained in the next chapter.

As 2009 draws to a close, the final tally is: 9 different doctors, 69 doctor visits, 12 tests and 1 surgery. Time for a new year and a new set of problems.

By the beginning of 2010, it has now been over 18 months since I have been able to work. Finances, to say the least, are pretty tough. A couple of friends of mine had approached me in the past about having a benefit for me. I didn't feel as though I should have one, because there are people out there worse off than me I said. I would much rather be on the other side helping them out. Denise, the main organizer, and my car saleswoman of all things, finally convinced me that BECAUSE of all the people I have helped that they in turn would now turn out to help me. She got in touch with Jackie who is my co-teacher at Sunday School, and they got the ball rolling. They set out to make this a memorable and profitable event. There were so many people from work and church that helped out, that each one had ideas of how to get things done. Friends and friends of friends helped out too. It would be impossible for me to name each and every one of them who helped, but to them I offer a HUGE "Thank You." Donations of food and prizes came in left and right. People donated paper products and tickets for entrance, door prizes and raffles. Everything was donated, so that meant that whatever funds were raised went directly to me to pay off my ever increasing medical expenses and household expenses as well. The local newspaper did a beautiful piece on my story, and I think that because so many people who read it recognized me from work, from the community or just knew me otherwise wanted to help. Folks I didn't even know donated money to me, and I made sure that each and every one of them who did got a personal thank you note from me. Some donated without giving their name, so I couldn't thank them personally, but please know that it was very much appreciated. Denise was right, people wanted to help me now in my time of need because of the many times I had done the same. I opened a special account with the funds, and it is used only for medical expenses. I had lost my medical benefits at work by this time, but was offered COBRA. I have since been paying that every month so that I don't lose any of the benefits I need.

As the year progressed again, the twitching got worse, the memory loss continued and the constant and chronic shortness of breath and fatigue continued as well. Climbing up the stairs was the worst. Not only were my feet in excruciating pain now, but I would have to stop 2 or 3 times just to get to the top. Walking to the mailbox became what seemed like a day trip, and things just continued to get worse. The neurologist ordered something called an EMG. This test is best described as being tasered! They take electric devices and zap your feet and legs to find out if there is any damage to your nerves or muscles. The electrical impulses measure the degree of that. Early Onset Parkinson's Disease?

My health continued a downward slide. I couldn't stand the pain in my feet and ankles anymore, and could barely walk in the morning. I just gave up on sleeping at night because the constant twitching and turning were driving me nuts. My family doctor finally ordered x-rays of my feet and ankles to see what was going on. The results came back that I had bone spurs and plantar fasciitis. Great, more problems and ANOTHER new doctor.

At about the same time as this, I learned my cardiologist was going on sabbatical, so this would be my last visit to her. Before I got to her, I had been told that I had another mild, silent heart attack. She said she wanted to share with me that I was one of her patients that she had doubts about being able to survive. She said, "When I first saw you, I thought to myself, this isn't going to end well. She's a young woman with so much to live for, and things don't look good for her." "I was wrong. You are a fighter and a very strong person." Now I had to find another cardiologist. I picked a local guy who I thought would be able to help me. I had been asked to send over all of my previous history before the appointment so that he could read over everything before he saw me. After keeping me waiting for what seemed like an eternity, he finally came into the exam room and asked "Why are you in my office?" I tried to tell him, but he wasn't paying attention because he was just flipping through the records I had sent over. Seems as though he never even looked at them before I came in. I was floored by what came out of his mouth. He said with an attitude, "None of this ever happened to you. It couldn't have because you don't fit the profile." He looked at me and said "I can't do anything for you. You don't need to come back." What? None of this ever happened? Perhaps if he had taken the time to actually read what was there instead of pretending to care and flip through the records, he would have seen that all of this did indeed happen regardless of whether or not I fit some sort of profile. Thanks for wasting my time. Oh yeah, you may want to work on your bedside manner. I walked out of there stunned and angry. Good riddance to you pal.

After getting the results of the x-rays, I went to a podiatrist. He sat there and listened to my history and took the time to look at the x-rays. He thought in light of all the other medical issues I had, it would be better off to start out with physical therapy rather than doing anything invasive. Sounds good to me! I started physical therapy in late November.

On a particularly busy Monday morning in early December, as I rushed out to go to the first of 3 doctor appointments for the day, I went to the garage to get in my car, and I twisted my ankle underneath of me when I missed the running board on the side of my car. I didn't give it a thought, because it didn't hurt at all. I actually had forgotten about it by the time I got to appointment #3 which was physical therapy. When I took my sneaker off, my ankle just exploded with swelling. The physical therapist took a look at it and said that I might want to have it looked at. Of course now that the sneaker was off, it wouldn't go back on. I ended up having to see doctor #4 that night, via an unplanned visit to a local urgent care. When they took an x-ray of the foot and ankle, it showed that I had torn all the ligaments in my ankle. The doctor asked me if I needed a pair of crutches to go home on, and I told her no because I had a pair at home from previous mishaps. I left there hobbling to get home. I called the podiatrist to let them know what had happened, and he wanted to see me. After examining the damage, and knowing that I still had the severe twitching, he decided to put a hard cast from my toes to my knee. This was done to prevent any further damage from occurring due to the twitching. Just what I needed 2 ½ weeks before Christmas. I went back for a checkup a couple of days before Christmas, and he took the cast off and sent me for more x-rays. It was still pretty messed up, so he put on a boot that would immobilize it. It was kind of like a ski boot. It was not lightweight, so you could hear me coming a mile away. I still had to use the crutches because I couldn't put any pressure on the ankle. Merry Christmas!

That was it for 2010, and the year ended like this: 10 doctors, 44 doctor visits and 16 tests.

By January 31, 2011, I had already logged 8 doctor appointments and 2 tests. Not the way I wanted to start out the year, but I had learned that this year, like the previous 3, was going to be more of the same. The fatigue wouldn't quit, the memory loss was going strong, the severe shortness of breath, and the twitching had now spread to both of my arms. My eyes were getting worse at this point too. The pressure had begun to build, so that meant that I had to see the eye doctor more often than normal. I also started feeling just plain worn out and bad. I kept getting dizzy and lightheaded, and had a couple of episodes where I fell down. One of those times I fell was when I was getting out of bed to turn the ceiling fan off and I lost my balance, fell and heard a crack in my neck and back. It was the middle of the night, so I thought that if I could make it until morning I would see my family doctor instead of going to the emergency room. I did make it, and when they x-rayed my neck and back, they found nothing was broken, thank goodness, but I had bruised a couple of ribs. I couldn't breathe as it was, and now I have bruised ribs to make it even more difficult. As the symptoms got worse and worse, my hematologist did more tests. She did specialized urine tests and more blood work. Some of the tests came back elevated, and was attributed to the APS. She also thought it was time for the dreaded colonoscopy. The test itself is nothing major. It's the prep that's awful. Because of the risk of bleeding, I again had to be off my anticoagulants for the week. I began feeling worse and worse as the week progressed, but I knew it had to be done. The concoction they make you drink the day before the procedure leaves much to be desired. I must say though that it does get the intended results! The night before, the hospital called and told me that it would be done in the very late morning or early afternoon the following day. Great, more waiting. By the morning of the procedure, I was so weak that I didn't know if I was going to make it. Keith had made the statement that he thought I would end up in the ER rather than the OR. I finally went to the hospital to check in, and they told me that my doctor had an emergency, so the test would be pushed back another hour. UGGHH! The test was finally done, and thankfully there was nothing wrong. I don't have to go through that again for another 5 years.

By March, I was still dealing with the daily dizziness and lightheadedness and some hearing loss in my left ear. The ENT ordered a test called a VNG which checks how well your eyes and ears work together. They put goggles on you and cover one eye. They then watch to see how well your eyes move to follow different lights and patterns at different speeds. They also shift you to different positions to see if you have something called positional vertigo. Hot and cold air is placed in your ears and it measures I believe, the pressures in your ears. I did have the positional vertigo. My right eye and left ear were not working properly together, so that gave me the feeling of being dizzy all the time. The VNG was repeated in June, and he recommended vestibular therapy to help regain my balance. I did that for a bit, but didn't notice much difference so I stopped. To date, I am still having the same issues with it.

August came, and it was time for another DEXA scan. I had that done and thankfully there are no major changes in the bone density.

The 2011 count, through October when this was written is 8 doctors, 41 doctor visits and 10 tests. There are still a couple of months left, so who knows what's in store!

9. The Social Security Nightmare

In the previous chapters, you have learned about my medical issues. Let me tell you a little bit about my job in this chapter.

I began working as a pharmacy technician in 1989. I became the first Certified Pharmacy Technician (CPhT) in my company in 1997. I had worked in the store closest to my home from 1989 until 2004. I then went to another one of our stores in 2004 and have been there ever since. For those of you who think that all we have to do in the pharmacy is slap a label on the bottle and throw some pills in, let me explain what other things go into filling your prescription. First, we have to be able to read the doctors handwriting. This is no easy task sometimes! We have to make sure that the prescription is written for the correct person. Have you had prescriptions here before for yourself? Yes, I understand that your child has, but we need your information to fill it for YOU. Make sure that strength and those directions are right, if not we have to call the doc and verify what they want. Quantity? That's got to be enough too. Oh, and did you mean to write for 100 of this narcotic or did you only write 10 and the patient or someone else changed it? Is there is a question about the number of refills? Verify it. How about the fact that you put the drug name down, but it comes in tablets, capsules or perhaps it's a cream vs. lotion vs. gel item? Wait! There's more! The insurance company will only pay for a generic version of medication, but this one doesn't come that way. Do you want to change the medication itself to make the insurance company happy or would you rather have the patient pay for what you actually wrote for? You are down here on vacation and forgot your "little white, round pill." Do you know the name of it? How about what it's for? Do you know where you had it filled and your doctor's name and phone number? All of these things plus many, many more things happen day in and day out without you ever knowing about them. We take the brunt of the anger if something goes wrong, but we are just doing our job to ensure that you get exactly what the doctor wants with the accuracy that has to be there. Would you rather we just "slap a label on it" and give you the wrong medication or would you rather leave there knowing that you have the correct medication that will help you the way it was intended to? Please think about this the next time you are told that it is going to take some time to fill the prescription. We can literally have your life in our hands if there is a mistake. As you can see, being in the pharmacy profession is a very rewarding, but stressful job. The amount of knowledge and accuracy that is involved is crucial for everyone. I no longer am able to accurately do my job and I am seen as a liability to the position because of all of the medical issues I have endured. I am no longer able to stand for long periods of time, cannot decipher the doctor's handwriting, have difficulty hearing on the phone, and most importantly, I can no longer do calculations or remember what the majority of medications are for. This could be a very deadly combination if I mistakenly give someone the wrong medication.

Do you see why I am unable to do my job? As for working somewhere else or doing something else, for the reasons I have already gone into, I am unable to work at all. Anyone who knows me knows my work ethic. I started working when I was young by selling that weekly newspaper. I then got my first real job in retail at age 16. I worked as a low level manager at a local retail chain for a couple of years before I started my career in the pharmacy. I have always worked and worked hard at what I do to be the best that I can. I hate the fact that I am unable to contribute any longer. People may question how I can do this book and remember the facts presented here. The reason is because I write everything down now. After the stroke, I realized that things were going to be very different for me. I decided that to help me remember and do day to day tasks that I would need to keep a record of what needed to be done. I literally at this point can turn around and forget what I was going to do. Move from one room to another, and I will have no recollection whatsoever of ever having the thought. My cognitive abilities are gone. I sometimes can't get the words or ideas from my brain to my mouth. This frustrates me. The physical limitations like the constant pain in my feet and legs, the extreme exhaustion and general feeling of sickness on a daily basis is hard for me to accept. I just keep going, hoping that one day I will get the help that I desperately need.

Social Security, on the other hand, does not seem to think I am disabled at all. As per their rules, you must be disabled for 12 months or longer before you can apply for benefits. Being the person that I am, I follow the rules and wait for that initial year to come. I fill out the mounds of paperwork that they make you do just to apply for the first time. It states that you will have a decision within 120 days after filing. I wait. On August 5, 2009, I get the first denial letter. It says that there is not enough evidence to approve me. I also get turned down for Supplemental Social Security Income (SSI) because I am told that Keith makes too much money. I don't quite understand how this works, as I am the one applying, not him. Ok, strike one. Everyone I speak to tells me that 99% of people who apply get turned down at first. They advise me to reapply. I do, and again, I wait. In the meantime, I continue to get Social Security statements in the mail saying that if I were to become disabled right now, then I would be eligible for x amount of dollars per month! This only further irritates me. A few weeks later, I get another denial letter. Strike 2. At this point, I call Social Security to see what I need to do next. I am told by one of the workers there that I can file a NEW claim. I do this right away. What the worker neglected to tell me was that once you file a new claim, the old one becomes null and void. I guess that's how they get around paying out benefits. By filing the new claim, Social Security will now only look back to May 2009 instead of May 2008. I lose a whole year off of my claim because of that misinformation I received. That means a whole year of pay that is gone forever. I am so furious about the whole thing that I contact my Senator. He gets in touch with Social Security, and they basically give him the runaround about it and ultimately tell him there's not enough evidence to support a claim. I am still waiting for the answer on the new filing, and low and behold, in October I get the denial letter. Strike 3. The reasoning in this letter is absurd, and inaccurate. Here is just a sampling of reasons I was given for being denied again.

"We have determined that your condition does not keep you from working because:" 1.You have Anti-Social & Syndrome (What does that even mean? It certainly doesn't make sense), 2. You had a stroke but can move your arms and legs, 3.You suffer from a blood condition, but lab work says you can work (really? Didn't know blood work could tell you that!), 4. You have lost the sight in one eye, but you have another one that should allow you to work, 5. You have a bone infection, but it is not severe and will heal with therapy (not one doctor has even suggested THAT one to me!), and 6. You have pain, but you can move your limbs (OK?). The closing statement is great too "If your condition gets worse and keeps you from working, call or visit any Social Security office. They work for your state but used our rules." Nice.

At this point, I figure it's time for a lawyer since I obviously don't have a snowball's chance for help. As I walk into his office, he looks at me and tells me that he can see that I genuinely need help. I give him all my previous medical records and denial letters, including the one the Senator received. He says he is not surprised. He also walks me through what needs to be done and we file a reconsideration request. The fourth request is now on its way to Social Security. Keep in mind that this is October 2010 when the appeal gets filed. Right there in black in white, it says that an appeal will take up to 120 days. This is key. Up to 120 days. We wait, and wait, and wait. It is now February 2011. I call my lawyer and he tells me he hasn't heard anything yet. I call Social Security's main number to see why. They tell me that the local office has just filed the claim to them on February 24th! It has been five months and they are just now filing it? I called my lawyer and needless to say, neither he nor I are happy at this point. I called the local office, and what I am told next really made my blood boil (no pun intended). Seems as though my request had been sitting on someone's desk since October. She just now got around to looking at it and filing it with the federal office. When I asked the person on the phone if there was anything they could do to expedite the claim, they actually laughed at me and told me that they couldn't, and I'd have to wait another 120 days for the federal office to handle it now. I called my lawyer right after I hung up. He had his secretary call the local office, and it took her 3 days to get a human on the phone to speak to. They gave her the same story. Sorry, can't help. Too bad. My next call after the lawyer was to the federal office. The woman I spoke to there was very nice, and kept apologizing for the delay. She told me she would expedite the claim to a dire need status that way I would be put at the top of the list for hearing the claim. In addition, while I was on the phone with her, she got in touch with the local office to see why they had taken so long to file the claim. I sat down after the phone call, and wrote a letter to my Congressman this time. I explained to him in detail what I was going through, and how the local office had failed to file the claim in a timely manner. His office contacted Social Security for me.

The morning after the phone call to the federal office, the phone rang at 7 AM. It was the manager of the local office yelling at me wanting to know why I went over his head! I told him exactly why, and how his staff had treated me. I told him it was obvious that they were at fault and that because of that, they should have made an effort to fix their mistake. He really didn't like hearing what I had to say, but I didn't care at that point because they were at fault and failed in their duties to help someone in need. It was ironic that about 2 days after that conversation, I got a letter from Social Security saying that they had received my request for reconsideration and had filed the necessary forms. The problem here was that they weren't even smart enough to change the date on the letter. They had left the original date as October 2010 on it as the date they received it. Shortly thereafter, I got a letter from the Congressman. He had forwarded a copy of the letter he received from Social Security to me. It was the exact same letter that the Senator had received many months before. It gave the reasoning as not enough medical evidence to support a claim. At this point, I am still waiting for the official denial of the claim. Finally, in April 2011, I get the denial letter stating, "Not enough medical evidence to support a claim." Strike 4. Are you serious? All of my doctors have bent over backwards to send every little detail that Social Security has requested. They even sent over and above what was required. I guess the 1500+ pages of proof are not enough evidence to prove I can't work. My lawyer appeals to try to have my case heard by an administrative law judge. That is fine, except because the system is so flawed and backed up with requests, that it takes 12-14 months to even find out if you will get a hearing. If they approve it, then you have to wait several more months to get the actual hearing. At this point, we will be looking at almost 5 years since this whole thing started.

Please excuse me a moment while I give you my soapbox moment. I was born and raised in this country. I have worked for well over 25 years of my adult life, paying into a system that promises to help you when you are in need. I have lived a clean and honest life and have always helped those in need the best way I can. Why, in my time of need, can't I get the help that I have earned and have a right to receive? Please answer me that. It makes me angry to think of how some people, natural citizens or otherwise, try to bilk the system. Why are they permitted to come here and get free housing, free medical care, and Social Security which they have never even paid a dime into when I have worked so hard my entire life and can't get the same? I know some people may be offended by these statements, but I only speak the truth. I'll step down from the soapbox now.

As of October 2011, I am still waiting to hear if I will be able to have that hearing. I probably won't know for at least 6 more months though, so this is my story to date.

10. Never Give Up. And Some Final Thoughts

I never thought I would be the one in the position to ask for help, but now that I am, not being able to receive it is very disheartening. Do I like being disabled? No. I would love to be able to do the things that I could before all of this happened, but I can't. My diseases are incurable, and the devastating effects are life-long. The toll on both my body and mind has been grueling, but I know that I can't give up the fight. I feel as though I have been blessed to have had this journey. Yes, it is frustrating to know that I will never be well again, but at the same time it has caused me to look at life a little differently than I would have had I not been given all these challenges. God has a plan for me. I don't know what it is, but He certainly does. Maybe the plan was for me to write this book and help others to overcome their own adversities. Maybe it is something totally different. I don't know for sure, but what I do know for sure is that God is good. What I do know, is that I had to be strong for my son. I had to be here for him to help him grow and flourish. I have something that I tell Alex all the time. It is simply "no matter what." He knows that means many different things like I love him, I am here for him, and we will get through things together "no matter what."

My Mom was the most courageous and upbeat person I have ever met. I looked to her for strength throughout these trying times, even if it meant looking skyward. I know that she is still here to guide me. She never lost her faith, her hope or her humor throughout the many tragic events that took place. In her final days, she still believed that she would return to work and be well again. Sadly, that wasn't to be.

People don't realize what a difference a positive attitude really does make. I have been asked on occasion if I am mad at God or mad at humanity for what has happened to me. Why should I be? I can't change my genetics, I can't change what has happened, and to dwell on those things is pointless. I had no control over them, but what I do have control over is how I approach them. Using faith, hope, and humor has helped me get through it all. Life is a journey, and the way you choose to take that journey is entirely up to you. I choose to live life to the fullest, laugh when I can and grieve when I need to. My motto has always been "I will survive." It also means that I will never give up. No matter what.